You Can DO IT

FASTING

EASY FAT-BURNING TECHNIQUES FOR

optimum health

WEIGHT LOSS

AND

wellness

NEW YORK TIMES BESTSELLING AUTHOR

JASINDA WILDER

This book is dedicated to Karri:

My sister, my friend—thank you for always being my wog partner, my cooking buddy, and my best friend. I couldn't do it without you!

Contents

A Note from the Author

THIS BOOK REPRESENTS REAL-LIFE EXPERIENCE GAINED through my own personal health journey; these are stories from my real life, and there are things here that are deeply personal. This is not a medical book written by a medical professional, so if you're seeking professional medical advice, you should keep looking.

Some of my health practices may not be right for you. As I've said before, in my previous non-fiction books, please discuss all personal health issues with your medical professional. I repeat, I am not in any way, shape, or form a medical professional. Comments, suggestions, and advice contained herein is intended for inspirational and motivational purposes only, and does not constitute medical diagnosis or treatment.

I am simply a mom, wife, author, chronic health failure, and curious health investigator. I have been on a lifelong quest to become healthy, and the information I'm sharing in this book outlines my practical findings after using myself as a guinea pig. I've been successful and I want to share that success with the whole world.

I do believe from my personal research that Type 2 Diabetes

is completely and totally curable, and I am living proof that you can improve insulin resistance. I believe traditional medicine's response to this disease, and the disease of obesity, is failing us, and we owe it to ourselves and our kids to look for alternative curative options. We must do whatever we can to save our kids from a fate that can only end in pain, suffering, and premature death.

I encourage you to look through the list of additional reading materials shown in the back of this book. I think it will prove extremely helpful on your journey to healing your body. My prayer for you is that whatever path you take, you find a way to free yourself from the vicious cycle of disease, pain, and suffering. I believe we all write our own story, and that each day is a new page and a new opportunity to create the life we want. I hope that by sharing my own personal health experiences with you that you will gain some insights, knowledge, and inspiration to make positive changes in your own health.

If I can do it, YOU CAN DO IT!

All my love to you,

Jasinda Wilder
March 2018

"YOU CAN'T GO BACK AND CHANGE THE BEGINNING BUT YOU CAN START WHERE YOU ARE AND CHANGE THE ENDING."

—CS LEWIS

PART 1

Fasting 101

Introduction

WHEN I WAS PREGNANT WITH MY SIXTH CHILD MY BODY began speaking to me, but it wasn't just speaking, it was screaming: sugar was making me sick—sugar was *killing* me. I would eat breakfast and then attempt to take a shower. I would stand up and then have to sit back down. My head would spin and I would shake. My body was finally forcing me to listen to it after putting it through so many years of crazy diets, surgeries, shakes, pills, and potions. It took the worry of impending motherhood, trying to protect the little life inside of me, for me to finally listen. It was one of those come-to-Jesus moments, shaking me out of the decades of craziness and abuse of my body.

Who or what was the villain? What had caused all the scarring and damage? The answer was SUGAR! If anyone tries to tell you that sugar is good for you, slap them and tell them it was from me—there is absolutely *nothing* about sugar that is good for your body. In fact, I liken it to poison, and that is no exaggeration.

Those scary days when I was four months pregnant were

the days when my little life-saver baby demanded my attention, sending me on a health journey that led me to where I am now—healthy, happy, and strong. Three years later I'm still learning, still figuring things out, but I know I've changed my life for the better.

I promised you at the beginning of my first self-health book, *You Can Do It*, that we would do this together, and I meant it! In this book we'll remind ourselves about where we've been and where we're headed. So, sit back and relax as we explore our health together.

I promise it will be a fun ride.

NO BIG GIRL LEFT BEHIND!

Enough introduction…let's get into it!

Running for My Life

I DON'T REMEMBER EVER WEIGHING LESS THAN 200 POUNDS. I asked my mom about this recently and she thinks I may have been over 200 pounds by fourth grade. So, it never occurred to me that my goal weight would ever be less than that. Remember, I'm nearly six feet tall and I wear a size 12 women's shoe, so I'm a big girl, but even my doctor thought a good goal weight for me would be around 215 pounds. Yes, that would still put me in the overweight range, but after looking at my fat percentage we were cool with 215 as a nice, solid goal for me. That being said, I always maintained that I just wanted my body to end up where it wanted to be; I was done fighting with it. Even when one of the OG Wilder Way ladies suggested that with her 5'10" frame, 180 lbs would be a solid goal, I couldn't fathom my body at that weight. It just wasn't something I could picture, or even consider. Despite this, I kept my mind open and focused on improving my health.

AUTOPHAGY

I like to keep up on health trends, and stay abreast of new studies on health and nutrition. A relatively new advancement that really got me excited was autophagy.

I was always worried about the long-term effects of living with so much excess weight for so long, and what it was doing to my body. Would I get cancer? Would I have so much old fat that it would cause me long-term harm? These are issues I often thought about, because—let's be honest—my health history aside, being morbidly obese for most of your life doesn't exactly set you up for great health as you age—it's hard on your heart, lungs, and joints, and I had many nutritional issues as a result. I really wanted to find a way to reverse some of the damage the years of unhealthy living had done, and autophagy really seemed like something that would help me achieve that.

What is autophagy exactly? Well, it's essentially your body eating itself... your body becomes a zombie. I know, I know, that sounds horrible, but it's the layman's version of what happens on a cellular level. Fasting brings on autophagy, and it helps the body clear out all of the junk that builds up. Autophagy has been in the health spotlight very recently because the 2016 Nobel Prize in Medicine went to Dr. Yoshinori Ohsumi and his research of autophagy.

I'll have more on this later, but it really got me into a whole new world, which ultimately led me to the focus of this book: medical and therapeutic fasting.

Yes, the "f" word.

I want to be very clear—fasting wasn't something I was doing regularly prior to Easter of 2017; I had done a little fasting before, but it was always for spiritual and religious reasons rather than for my physical health.

When I began reading about and researching fasting for health, and specifically autophagy, at the beginning of 2017, I didn't really have the nerve to try it until Holy Week. Go figure! I guess I thought that since I already had some experience with religious fasting, Holy Week would be a good time to try fasting with the idea of initiating autophagy. I mean, if you can't fast for Jesus, who can you fast for? I figured I'd kill two birds with one stone, hopefully improving both my physical health *and* spiritual health at the same time. Sounds like a win-win scenario, right? I thought so.

That initial week of fasting led me on a fasting exploration, which really gave me some amazing insights into my health and my body. I discovered that healing the damage I'd done to my body wasn't just about putting good, nutritious food into my body, but it was also about giving my body a break from eating, letting some of that old fat and protein break down so I could really get "clean," and detox. I was seeing some great non-scale results, as well: I was starting to feel better, I was sleeping better, I had increased energy, and my skin was clearing up.

What if I could continue to heal my body through fasting? This was an intriguing question I asked myself and I knew I wanted to try it.

If you've lived like I have, where eating garbage all day

long was the norm, it can be difficult, when losing weight, to get that final fifteen to twenty pounds of fat to release. Why is that? Because it has been happily sitting in your body for the past ten, fifteen, twenty, or in my case thirty years! A doctor once told me my fat had the characteristics of dense tumors— this stuff just didn't want to leave!

The issue is that with some problem areas, this fat just won't disperse without employing very specific diet protocols such as fasting, among others.

There are even studies currently taking place showing that old, white, visceral fat won't *ever* leave unless you find a way to change its color to the easier-to-disperse brown fat.

After reading a lot of books and these new studies, and learning as much as I could, I chose to try fasting.

> WARNING: fasting isn't for everyone—I wouldn't recommend it for those with low body fat percentages, children, or pregnant or nursing women, but for most everyone else, it's really okay to do this from time to time.

Over the course of the last year, through periodic fasting, I've even seen my metabolism increase rather than decrease, as we are often told. In fact, I would say that since I started doing therapeutic fasting my overall health, strength, muscle tone, endurance, and body function have all improved. In addition, I have been able to work more efficiently and my mind is clearer.

As I became more convinced about the benefits of fasting,

something interesting happened to me. I applied the practice of fasting to other areas of my life, not just food—social media, negativity, alcohol; there is more on this later in the book, but the benefits of cutting something out of your life for a pre-determined period of time cannot be overstated.

Do you see why I just had to share this part of my health puzzle with you?

So...how do you incorporate fasting into the Wilder Way lifestyle? I'm so glad you asked!

In the following chapters you'll read about why I think incorporating fasting into your health regimen is the very best way to achieve long-term success in weight loss, but also in overall health and wellness. For me it has never been about looking better—I think I looked pretty decent before! For me, this is about FEELING GOOD, and living a long healthy life with my hot AF husband.

Are you with me?

How and Why I Fast

THERE ARE SO MANY DIFFERENT WAYS TO FAST AND, having tried them all, here's what I've learned: as long as you follow a few basic rules, you WILL be successful. The great thing about fasting is that you can make it fit whatever lifestyle works best for you. For me, as a mom, it's really important that I eat dinner with my family. My kids are sad if I don't eat with them. The way I work fasting into my life is simple: before I start a 24-hour fast I eat with my kids at dinnertime, and then twenty-four hours later I'm able to have dinner with them again.

There are a few exceptions to this; for example, if Jack and I are traveling, and the kids aren't with us, then that's a great time for us to do an extended fast.

> As a side note, I've found I actually feel much better when traveling if I'm not eating. Jack drives like a crazy man and you probably know air sickness is pretty common, so having an empty stomach is actually really great for me; I've never been car sick or had air sickness while doing an extended fast.

But I digress. What do I call an extended fast? For me, anything over a full twenty-four hours is an extended fast. 32, 48, 64, 72 hours are all common fasting intervals. Personally, I won't fast longer than five days because I don't want to chance incurring the possible health issues or problems that can be encountered beyond that point. Even when I fast for over three days I check my blood pressure and blood sugar regularly. And I use plain old common sense; if I don't feel well for any reason, I stop.

> If you do find you want to do a fast longer than five days, I strongly recommend you seek the assistance of a doctor who can monitor you.

I fast totally clean, and I fast completely at random depending on how I'm feeling. Clean fasting means I don't eat a single thing, and I usually only drink water. I fast this way to be sure I'm triggering the most effective autophagy.

Studies have shown if you really want to get the most bang out of your autophagy buck, then you need to stick to water and salt while fasting—more on that later, though. This means no other liquids, no gum, and no broth—nada, nothing! To quote my fasting friend Megan Ramos, "Water and salt and not another darn thing!"

I've been trying to tighten up my skin after significant weight loss, and for that reason getting the most from fasting was a high priority for me. If I can lose some of this skin without resorting to surgery, I want to do it. SIGN ME UP! Many of you have emailed me asking about skin-tightening products you've seen: I promise, if it's out there, I've probably tried it. The truth is, though, so much of our skin elasticity is due to plain old genetics and I've found that these products never live up to the hype. There are other factors, of course, that determine whether you will have loose skin or not including age, the speed at which your weight is gained or lost, and *how* you lose your weight.

I truly believe that keeping your blood sugar and insulin levels low and steady in combination with fasting is the way to go if you have loose, hanging skin. It might not be the most fun or dramatic, but it's the most effective method. Think about photos you've seen of people who are literally starved—and I mean concentration camp-level starved—do they ever have huge flaps of loose, hanging skin? No! That's because when your body eats your fat from itself, the skin goes with it. This might not be a pretty thing to talk about, but because I've had so many people ask me about this I think it's important to mention it here.

But back to the practicalities of fasting. I usually fast with plain water—sometimes carbonated water—and salt, and nothing else. My one variation is black coffee, because sometimes I just need my coffee!

Let me be very clear in saying I am *not* unique in that I often feel better physically when I'm in a fasted state versus when I'm not. I often have a better workout, a more productive day, and have more even energy. My very favorite fasts are twenty-four hours because they're just so easy now. I can eat an early dinner with my kids on a Sunday and then not eat again until dinner on Monday evening, and half of that fasting time is when I'm sleeping. EASY PEASY!

If you're new to fasting and just want to dip a toe in, I would suggest maybe trying a 24-hour fast. I've learned fasting is as much an exercise of the body as it is of the mind: but as you continue to fast, you'll find it does become easier.

> I've done many extended fasts now and only once have I ever felt the need to cut it short. It was during a very difficult, stressful time in my life, on top of which, it was that time of the month. I was about two days into my fast and my period started early, and I had a very strong headache coming on, so it just didn't make sense to continue fasting.

My husband is my number one lab rat, and he was a struggle pony with the 24-hour fasts for months. He would whine and cry until I would finally just beg him to eat. This went on for some time until finally, one day, he said, "Hey, I've gone thirty-two hours and that was totally easy. I wasn't even hungry!"

To many people, the thought of not eating for thirty-two hours straight is simply unfathomable. But if we think about it, it's only been in the last few decades that our relationship with food has undergone so many radical changes. Today we live in an era where food is in front of our faces all day long. We can't scroll through Facebook, walk to the bathroom, or drive down the street without images of food being pushed into our minds every waking moment.

Our primal ancestors didn't eat all day long. Sure, they thought about food a lot but that was because they were hunting and gathering food every day. Then they repeated the process all over again the next day. They didn't have a big breakfast of oatmeal or pancakes, and then follow it up with McDonald's for lunch, and pizza for dinner. Heck, they didn't even have a 1,000 calorie Starbucks in the middle of the day. Life was difficult and they didn't have the luxury of buying food in a grocery store

But we live in a different world now; it's a McWorld, but do you really want to be a McGirl? The McGirl lives a very different life than that of her primal sister, who spent the day walking, lifting, balancing, and moving. If I'm given a choice, I want to be the Primal Princess, not the McGirl with the big health problems to match her large exterior.

And again, let me point out, this has NOTHING to do with beauty—this has everything to do with living and dying. I don't want to die prematurely; I'm choosing to live a long and healthy life.

And, as crazy as it sounds, I believe my best life might just be the fasted life. It might be a life where I regularly spend twenty-four hours when food is the last thing on my mind. In my busy life, I can usually go until about 3 p.m. on a fast day without even thinking about food. To be honest, considering that for thirty-six years food was the first and sometimes only thing on my mind, it's a welcome change not to be continually thinking about food.

Of course, there are weeks on end when I'm in no mood to fast, so I don't. For example, there was a month last summer when I took a big old fasting break. My body was screaming for a little variety so I changed things up. I really believe much of my success with my continued health improvement and weight loss is due to the fact that I'm constantly changing what I'm doing, so my body isn't adapting to any one thing for too long. I might do a full week of all black plates followed by twenty-four to forty-eight hours of fasting that I then break with a nice white plate breakfast of baked oatmeal and berries. My body is like WHHHHHHAAT? But my blood sugars stay stable, I have *so much* energy, and I don't have the long-term and sometimes scary side effects of someone who only does low carb or keto all the time.

Fasting is working for me. My hormones thank me. My body is healthy and happy. Life is good.

For someone who isn't really in tune with their body this might sound kind of complicated. But when you're listening to your body it's easy to know when you need carbs, or fats, or more food, or less food. And, no, this has nothing to do with that old, failed notion of calorie restriction.

We've all been there, done that, and bought the t-shirts. But why do we continue to do the things that never work or never last? I recently talked to someone who told me they were doing Weight Watchers for the seventeenth time! To me, this is just plain insanity—what will happen this time to make it any different from the other sixteen times? Come on! There is a better way to take control of your health.

Now might be the time for you to try something new, something different. If you have excess weight you want to get rid of, use your body's natural, internal processes to burn that fat. The goal is to become so in tune with your body that you know exactly what it needs and when it needs it.

> These are the ways that I've found always promote fat loss:
> 1) Eat your fats together
> 2) Eat your carbs together
> 3) Move your body
> 4) FAST!

This has been my exact experience. I promise if you do these things, the fat will melt right off your body. In fact, I'm so sure I will bet you a RUNNING SUCKS t-shirt on it!

At this point in my journey, I don't even pre-plan my meals anymore; I just make what I feel like when I want it. When I'm really feeling satiated and full, I don't eat, or sometimes I just don't feel like eating breakfast or lunch, while there are other weeks when I need three full meals a day plus snacks. It's much easier for me to begin fasting after a few days of eating only black plates because, after a few days of that, fasting just feels natural. I now know just what my body needs, and when I need to it.

> When I'm engaged in social activities where my family or friends are eating, I naturally feel like I should eat with them and I never deprive myself of that. I now know how to manage my body and my life so that nothing is lost.

I know you might be reading this thinking I'm crazy, but you too can get to a point where your body will be happily content being fueled by the fat sitting there since you ate that whole bag of Cheetos in 1986. True story!

Before we get to the practicalities and how-tos of fasting, I want to leave you with a list of the other great benefits you can get from fasting:

- CHANGE IN BODY COMPOSITION: fasting works on all the "problem areas" and increases human growth hormones for building muscle and burning fat

- BOOSTS METABOLISM: good for stubborn stalls

- IMPROVES INSULIN SENSITIVITY and NORMAL-IZES/LOWERS BLOOD SUGAR

- HELPS WITH INFLAMMATION and IMMUNITY: balances hormones and generates free radicals

- PROTECTS THE BRAIN FUNCTIONS

- IMPROVES THE HEART and NORMALIZES BLOOD PRESSURE

- IMPROVES SKIN QUALITY

- PROMOTES LONGEVITY

PART 2

Getting Started

The Wilder Way 3.0

THE HARDEST PART OF TRYING SOMETHING NEW IS ALWAYS getting started, so let's just jump right in with a few general notes.

First, the optimal time to begin your fast would be right after you've had a few days of really fatty black plates—this gets your body prepped for fat burning.

Second, don't tell people you're going to fast. Obviously, it will be difficult to hide it from a spouse or other close family members, but don't make a public announcement or start a Go Fund Me page saying that you're planning to stop eating; THIS WILL NOT GO WELL. Just be a chill faster.

Third, always have water with you. I like to have bubbles in my water because it causes me to drink more slowly.

Fourth, keep salt with you at all times; I like the pink chunky salt from Amazon. If you feel as if you want to eat, have a pinch of salt and then drink some water.

I recently read an awesome book about how badly we all need minerals and salt; so don't be scared of it! Our bodies were made for salt and it will pass through you quickly if you're drinking a lot of water. Repeat after me, S-O-S: SUCK ON SALT! Salt is also great for when you're running, but more on that later on. Just try to have salt with you when you are fasting so you don't get into a situation where you feel yucky because your electrolytes are off and you don't have salt handy.

The best way to get your feet wet with fasting is by simply skipping breakfast; this gets your fasting muscle flexing. My Wilder Way Eight-Week Fasting Challenge starts you off by skipping breakfast and replacing it with water, coffee, or tea—that's just *one* meal each day you don't eat. I like to start by skipping breakfast because adding your hours of sleep on top of the time you're fasting gives you great results.

Please, don't overwhelm yourself, and give yourself grace. This is all about learning, and you will get there if you just keep trying.

THE EIGHT-WEEK FASTING CHALLENGE

WEEKS ONE AND TWO

Prep your body to fast by eating heavy, fatted black plates for a few days. These foods would include things like eggs, bacon, avocado, heavy cream, dark chocolate, oil, and butter. Can you hear me singing "These are a few of my favorite things?" I am! Make sure to include these heavy fat items in your black plate menus. The weekend before you begin your fast is a great time to enjoy your black plate meals. Who doesn't love an avocado- and cheese-filled omelet cooked in butter or oil with a side of bacon for Saturday or Sunday breakfast? Then, make sure you have something really satisfying the evening before your fast—dark chocolate might be a good choice, or some heavy whipping cream with berries.

Then, the next day, on Day 1 of your fast, begin with just water and coffee or tea, but don't add anything to your coffee, water, or tea—no sugar, no milk or cream, no flavoring, nothing! You want to make sure you're fasting clean to get the very best results! You can then go ahead and eat your white or black plate lunch, dinner, and snack as you normally would for two full weeks. It's as easy as that!

I will say I've found white plates are better for breaking my fast, while I like to make sure my last meal or snack is something black because it gives me a fuller and more satisfied feeling going into the fast. It's really important you test things out for yourself and see what works best for your body. I've found some people even sleep better with some good carbs before bed—if you're one of those people, don't worry, you will be okay! I find that I might just need more water or salt the next day as I get into my fast. It might be a touch harder for some, but not impossible.

> Three things I'm going to repeat over and over: 1. it is natural to feel a peak of hunger, but it does get easier; 2. if you don't feel well, stop your fast; and 3. JOURNAL, JOURNAL, JOURNAL!

WEEKS THREE AND FOUR

We're going to kick it up a notch, now—try to skip both break-fast *and* lunch! I know, I know, I'm BATSHIT CRAZY! But when you start to see results and start feeling better, it will be easier than you could even imagine. Here's the kicker: you can eat as much as you want with dinner and before you go to bed—this is called One Meal a Day (referred to hereafter as OMAD) style fasting, and even having a decent-sized snack within your eating window is totally okay! Go for it! You may find you aren't even all that hungry after a large dinner and you will want to skip an after-dinner snack and that's okay too! As usual, we're going to listen to our bodies, which means some days we might need more food than others.

WEEKS FIVE AND SIX

I want you to try OMAD in a short eating window. Sometimes I do a few hours and sometimes I might keep it open a full hour. It is also important to note that most days I stick to carb cycling, but I'm always mixing it up and I'm always listening to my body, and when I feel myself needing carbs, I eat carbs. I believe this is usually connected to my hormones and my cy-cle, but I've learned now in my thirty-eight years not to fight my body when it's screaming for something because it's almost always screaming for a reason. Now, I have on occasion tried to stick to black plates during the week because that's just what feels best and then I "carb up" on the weekends, which for me are more freestyle because I really want to enjoy them with my family. If my family is going to a special event or wants to get some gluten-free pizza and Halo Top for a birthday, I'm not going to sweat it. You know from my previous books that I am not at all about deprivation or being left out—if I want to join in and enjoy, I DO!

WEEKS SEVEN AND 8

I want you to experiment with whatever feels good for you. Some people might want to try a 24, 36, or 72-hour fast, while other people might want to go back to a week of black plates because their bodies feel a bit burnt out from the intermittent or window fasting. Just like my previous challenges, this is when I really want you to dial in and decide what you feel is best for you. I personally think that as long as your body is in the overweight, obese, or morbidly obese classification, and you're neither a child nor pregnant or breastfeeding that fasting for a few days is safe for *almost everyone*. Please consult with your doctor if you have any specific concerns, but quite honestly people have been fasting for religious reasons since the dawn of time. It is only more recently that we've stopped practicing a life of fasting, even though we're always feasting in our American culture. There is a lot of great evidence that a 3-day fast can totally reset your body, specifically your immune system.

I would suggest even someone with a healthy BMI could benefit from a 3-day fast on a quarterly basis. A 3-day fast is a really good sweet spot for people—you usually feel pretty darn good by day three. Beware of hours 18-20, though, as they're usually the hardest, because that's when hunger peaks. Once you get past that stretch, though, most people are golden. It really does give your body a break and the health benefits far outweigh the missed meals.

> After completing all eight weeks, it is important to continue to journal, and to listen to your body.

The amazing thing I've found through my own fasting is that I have so much more time. In the morning I just grab my coffee and get to work, which also gives me some time to do things I don't otherwise have time for. I've discovered having ten to fifteen minutes of quiet time is vital to me. Whether I'm journaling, praying, or just sitting, this time really helps me clue into what my mind, body, and soul need. I'll have more on this later.

It is always totally okay to change your plans. I have a great example of this from my own experiences. I said earlier I find it much easier to fast while traveling—my lifelong car and air sickness completely go away when my stomach is empty, so when I know I'm going to be in a car or airplane for a long period of time, I plan to fast while in transit and then eat again when we arrive. Because we live hours from a major airport, this is usually a 24- to 48-hour fast.

Well, on a recent trip with my daughter, I decided since we were going to be so busy with her classes and workshops that I would just fast until we got home. It was a long weekend and we were coming off holiday feasting, so it just seemed like a good idea. When we got to our hotel my daughter said she REALLY wanted us to have a special dinner together, and she wanted *steak*! How could I say no to that? She's my oldest daughter and we honestly don't get many chances to get away for a weekend like this, so after thinking about it I decided a big juicy steak with my beautiful and excited daughter was an even better idea than fasting. She was really happy, and we even enjoyed some Halo Top ice cream after our steak.

I'm totally able to control these things now, when for most of my life I felt like they controlled me. The other thing I think is really important to point out is that this is a process—fasting is a muscle. In all things I think it's important to give yourself grace. I didn't start fasting at all until I was three years into my health journey and quite honestly I'm not sure what my results would have been if I tried it at the beginning. I think easing into this gradually and in logical steps has made it so much easier for me; I haven't been in a rush, but have continued to take it step by step, always letting my body lead me.

I also still think that as a diet-based society, we push our bodies in ways that don't produce the results we want because our bodies push right back. Lose sixty pounds in two months on a liquid diet and watch yourself gain back eighty pounds once you start eating again—I've seen this happen over and over again. Balance is absolutely vital in life. Which is another thing that really spoke to me about feasting and fasting. For one thing, it just works well with my personality and lifestyle, but now, almost a year into doing all sorts of fasting, I can honestly say my ability to let my body heal itself on its own terms has been amazing, not only for my body but also for my mind.

So take the time. Give yourself constant grace. Wake up each day focused on your self-worth, and if you fail, start again.

A Fasting Experiment

As I mentioned before, I've water fasted for spiritual reasons a few times in my life, usually during a "lock-in" type thing during high school when we were raising money for hungry people in the world. Typically, these fasts lasted around twenty-four to thirty-six hours. In retrospect, the hardest part about those fasts was the mind game I played prior to doing it. I was sixteen years old and weighed 300 lbs, but had so much anxiety thinking I would starve to death. So, before the fast, I would eat a whole pizza and half a cake. True story! Safe to say I wasn't totally in touch with reality at sixteen.

Loading up with all those carbs may have not been the smartest thing, because over those twenty-four hours it really did feel like I was actually starving. We were allowed to have juice, which of course only made it that much worse. It was a slow, painful experience for my poor sixteen-year-old body! I was such a mess, guys! I'm so glad you didn't know me then, and if you're reading this and you did know me then, I sincerely apologize.

My point here is to tell you that until I had my third son, and read an amazing, eye-opening book on fasting for spiritual reasons, my history with fasting was extremely sketchy at best. When I read that book, I think I did a few fasts that lasted only a few days at most, and I had broth and liquids during them, so in my mind it wasn't a very clean fast. I don't remember it being all that hard physically, but it was difficult for me mentally.

Then, when I started fasting seriously last year, I began by skipping meals here and there with no spiritual component to it. I was really focused on the health benefits and not so much the spiritual side of things. My first real extended fast was not only for health reasons, but also for my mental and spiritual well-being.

It's an odd phenomenon, perhaps, but fasting slows the world down for me. When I turn my attention away from eating, my whole world just slows down and relaxes. I have more time. I have more focus. There's more time for my prayer life and my journaling. There's self-reflection and quiet, which is much harder for me to find time for when I'm eating. I can't really explain how or why this is, it just is.

Some of the weeks I remember the most vividly over the past year were also the weeks when I was fasting. To me, this is just further proof that my brain was clearer and functioning more efficiently. And since I knew I would probably write a book on this practice, it's great I'm able to recall these things so easily. The other really cool thing about those weeks of fasting is that I was at my most productive.

Not only did I have all this extra time, but the time I had was really great for my work life and my home life: I was organizing, I had time for a bath, I went for a walk with my husband, and my daily word count went up! Bonus, bonus, bonus! The other really funny thing about my first extended fast is everyone—and I mean everyone—told me how great I looked. I call it the fasting "glow and float" because there's some sort of glow that comes from fasting which makes people notice you, and your body actually feels physically lighter. I think the feeling of lightness mostly comes from not having much poop in your gut, but it's also something more ethereal, something that just makes you feel…different.

I don't recall ever feeling that way at any other time in my life, and I promise that I have NEVER had so many people tell me I look good than when I'm three to five days into an extended fast. Again, it's something you just have to experience yourself to fully understand, but the "glow and float" phenomenon is real. BONUS!

I particularly like to fast when approaching a spiritual season, or a season of celebration. When I know there's a special time coming up, I like to give my body some downtime, either before or after. But don't get me wrong, I fully embrace the idea of a feasting and fasting balance in life, and when I feast, I feast—hello, bacon and dark chocolate!

Before Christmas last year, I knew I needed to slow down, spend time meditating on joy, the gifts of the season, and family. For me, fasting was the perfect way to do this—unplug from food for a while and deeply, intentionally focus on these things leading up to the holiday season, and then celebrate with my family with our traditional Christmas Eve dinner. Great idea, right? I thought so.

Of course, as with anything I make grand plans for, life threw a wrench at me. Our family faced one difficulty on top of another for the entire month of December. I was involved in a situation with a drunk driver that resulted in a fatality—understandably, that really shook me up. My kids were sick, we had work setbacks, my kids were sick again...and by the time we got to the final weeks before Christmas, I was just worn down. I could very easily have decided fasting was just going to make things worse and changed my plan entirely, but I didn't. The reason I'm saying this isn't to make you feel like I'm some sort of fasting superhero, but to say that sometimes stress equals eating for me.

I decided that eating might only add more stress for me when I really needed more peace, and you know something? That's truly what it did for me. I can't say it would be the same for you, or that I'll even make the same decision next year, but my experience was amazing. So amazing, in fact, that even my kids said I was the least stressed and most joyful they'd ever seen me during a holiday season. I wasn't the frazzled holiday mama I usually am. Not only that, but the things I'd anticipated being difficult and challenging just weren't that hard at all. It's largely a head game, I've realized.

Our annual holiday cookie and baking day fell during that fast, and guess what? I did my baking while fasting! Now, this *was* challenging because I couldn't taste anything, and if you know me at all, you know I literally cook and bake everything by taste…to the point that I'm usually not hungry by the time the food is done because I've eaten so much already.

We also host a small get-together at our house each year on the last day of school before the holiday break, for the families of my kids' school friends. When I throw a party, the main event is food. Guess what? I was right smack dab in the middle of my extended fast on the day of the party. What was I going to do? Well, did something I've never done as a party hostess: I spread out all the beautiful food and focused exclusively on my guests. I didn't have a sip of wine, a morsel of cheese, or a single holiday cookie. This gave me the opportunity to chat with, hug, and interact with the people we'd opened our house to.

When we host anything, the party, the people, and the whole event often goes by in a blur. This party was totally different. I can remember details of every moment, and I can recall the conversations I had with each person. The kids had a really special ornament exchange with their friends which, to be totally honest, I'm not sure I would've been able to sit and watch had I been rushing around trying to eat and drink while hosting. There's absolutely nothing I would change about that evening. It was just so cool to just focus on things other than food.

For some, this might not seem like anything very unique, but for me—someone who was ruled by food for most of her life—getting through that party without even thinking about food and, instead, focusing on the guests? That was something of a marathon accomplishment. And let me just pat myself on the back a little, because that food looked AMAZING! If you're on my Instagram you might have seen it: cheese, meat, beautiful grapes, wine, #wilderway cheesecakes, and cookies. It was glorious. And I didn't really miss having any of it. I mean, I'm sure it was tasty, but I was so busy spending time with our guests and focused on celebrating the season with my family and friends that it was almost too easy.

My fasting muscle was flexing.

I also think the stars aligned for me with this spiritual fast leading into Christmas. The year before last, my family experienced a tragedy on Christmas Eve and I had so much fear and anxiety about what had taken place that I really needed to do something radical to be able to enjoy the season this year. Yes, this fast was radical, but I think it definitely helped me get through what could have been a difficult season. So get radical! If you've experienced times when you feel things are flying by too fast, maybe that's God calling on you to slow it down.

I'm so grateful for the times I had that week with God, my family, and my friends. Life can move like a freight train, and I think there's a very real need for all of us to create space in our lives for both feasting and fasting, for celebration and silence, for periods of waiting, and the joy of indulgence.

As I've mentioned several times already, your fast won't work the same for you as it does for me, but one thing that is similar for all of us is that how we feel, how we approach our wellness journey can and does change from week to week. This is why I believe journaling during your fasting times is so important. In those quiet, radical moments you'll realize things which will be life-changing. I promise.

You can do it!

Fasting From Diets

(WARNING: RANT AHEAD!)

diet: to restrict oneself to small amounts or special kinds of food in order to lose weight.; "It's difficult to diet"

Synonyms: To be on a diet, eat sparingly; to lose weight, watch one's weight, reduce, slenderize; crash-diet; "she dieted for most of her life."

life·style: the way in which a person or group lives; "the benefits of a healthy lifestyle."

Synonyms: way of life, way of living, life, situation, fate, lot.

Can we all please just agree to *stop* dieting?

Haven't we had enough, already?

Did the fad grapefruit diets of the 80s teach us nothing?

When I scroll through my Facebook feed, all I see is post

after post about the newest shake or quick-fix pill, or how many points there are in this recipe, or how many ketones are contained in this supplement, or how hard we have to scrub ourselves with a special fat-blaster stick before the pounds melt off.

I speak from experience when I say I know how hard it is to find something that will work for you, but unless you're willing and able to commit to your diet of choice from now until forever, none of that will ever be anything except a temporary Band-Aid solution. Diets only address a symptom and ignore the most important underlying issues, which cause things like diabetes and heart disease.

There is one truth when it comes to eating and wellness and that is this: science has known this for a long time, but the truth is covered up by the multibillion-dollar food industry: it's the sugar and carbs that make us fat and unhealthy, not dietary fats. Yes, I said it, and you can quote me—put it on my tombstone: *Here lies Jasinda Wilder, who did NOT die from eating fats.*

The truth is, for many of us who are overweight, fat is still a really difficult topic. We have so much fear about eating fat that we feel compelled to cross our fingers and say a prayer before eating every piece of bacon that goes in our mouth. We've been told for decades that fat was the bad guy, but the plain, scientific truth is…it's not. Fat was always our friend; it just got a bad rap. Now, years after science has very clearly proven it actually isn't fat that makes us fat, we're still scared of it.

So what are we doing? We still try to "diet" by lowering

our fats and increasing our carbs and sugars to compensate. The truth is, body composition is all about hormones. I'm sure you've heard people say, "a calorie is a calorie." Well…a calorie is not a calorie; calories just aren't the same once they're inside the body. You can eat fifty calories via one donut hole, or fifty calories in two cups of broccoli—if you think your body is going to process those two very different versions of fifty calories the same way, you're just plain wrong. The broccoli is dense with nutrients, vitamins, fiber; the donut is nothing but sugar and carbohydrates. The broccoli will give you fuel, whereas the donut will end up on your backside and stay there.

Sure it would be great if things were different, but they aren't. Our bodies are much more complex, and it's the nutritional value of calories that matters to our biology and our well-being.

Our insulin levels rise when we eat anything, but how high it rises and how long it stays there is what determines how fat burns and how it stays in the body. When you have lots of insulin in your body, very little fat is going to burn. In this day and age when we're *always* eating, and often eating foods that cause insulin to not only rise but also to *skyrocket*, it's only common sense that most of us are struggling to lose weight no matter what we do. And that will always be the case until we get that insulin under control. The way the average American eats means insulin levels are always heightened, and if we can't lower our insulin levels and learn to keep them low, the result is diabetes, heart disease, cancer, autoimmune disease, inflammatory issues, Alzheimer's, and other neurological issues. We know this to be true, and there are *so many* studies which have shown and continue to show us this truth, yet many of us are still not getting the message.

Don't believe me? *PLEASE* read Dr. Jason Fung's amazing blog, and look at the results he's had with reversing Type 2 diabetes; also take a look at the research by Dr. Benjamin Bikman at BYU, and read the *Metabolic Approach to Cancer* by Dr. Nasha Winters (I'll list more in the additional resources section of the book).

The most important factor in making a decision about what to do about your weight and wellness, and why to do it, is to consider how long you think you'll be able to maintain that plan. How long can you keep up with the way you're living, eating, and moving? If you're miserable and unhappy, you'll probably not be able to last very long. If you're really motivated, *maybe* you'll last for six months to a year. The frustrating thing is that when we get close to our weight-loss goals we often begin to sneak unhealthy things back into our diet. When that happens it doesn't take long until we're back where we started, and then some.

Diets don't work.

A diet is inherently temporary; a diet is something that, for most of us, triggers an intensely negative connotation. What we need to do to be successful at losing weight and keeping it off is making a *lifestyle* change—I preached this in my first two nonfiction books, *You Can Do It* and *You Can Do It: Strength*. We have to get to the point where we can say we're *done* with how we've been living, and then make the decision that we want to live a different way *FOREVER*. You have to decide you *WILL NOT* go back to those old, unhealthy habits, *no matter what.*

A new lifestyle means a new way of living—making long-term changes for the better. With most people, I see this happening when they've either seen someone die because of bad health, or because they themselves got a frightening diagnosis, or some other big turning point in life made them want to totally uproot the "diet" mentality for something they can be successful at and maintain.

> Making a lifestyle change rarely happens quickly or easily, but once you've made the changes you'll have trouble believing it took you so long.

Something else I've noticed is that making lifestyle changes frequently takes a few rough starts before it really sticks. People think they're in that place only to find out that they really aren't ready yet for true, lasting, drastic change. In my groups I often see people take two or three attempts before everything clicks into place, where they're really in the mental space to make the necessary changes for a new lifestyle.

A lifestyle is something you stick to, no matter what. It becomes part of the way you live your life day in and day out, so when things pop up which would ordinarily throw you off on a diet, your lifestyle will still remain intact. You've created an environment where you can allow yourself grace, freedom, and satisfaction. If you're on a diet, failure is inevitable because there is no tolerance for any misstep from your plan. You don't want to continue because you've been defeated by too many mistakes.

A lifestyle gives something to you, whereas a diet takes things away—it's all how you look at it. You make mistakes, you stumble, you have setbacks, but since you know this is just the way you live, you focus on making better choices the next meal or the next day. There's no guilt or shame with a lifestyle, because it's part of what's expected. Life happens and no one is perfect, but this is now part of how you live, and you take the challenges and setbacks in stride and move on to the next opportunity. With a lifestyle, you don't have to make a social media post explaining that you fell off your diet, because it won't be a Facebook-worthy status. You do your thing and you carry on with the way you live because that's the way you live, it's just the way you roll.

> Once we get out of the ridiculous mindset that our journey to health and wellness is some sort of game show where the loser gets voted off the island, we can be even more successful.

As I said in my previous books, if someone had told me it would take me as long as it has to be where I am, I would have laughed and looked for some other way. But now I've seen how the slow and steady changes add up, how I'm not deprived of good food, how I wake up with energy and feel good every day, how my skin glows, how great my test results are, and how I was able to have my medical port removed after almost ten years, I would have committed to this lifestyle even if it took twice as long!

When you change your lifestyle, you accept that there's no other way to be. You slowly make positive changes over the course of months and years, rather than thinking in terms of weeks. It's part of your life rhythm.

When people ask Jack how he ran a marathon, he says one step at a time, and that's exactly how this race is run, too: one little step at a time, one day at a time, and one meal at a time.

Fasting from Alcohol

Before I started fasting, I didn't realize how much I depended on a drink with dinner, or a drink or two after dinner. It often becomes a gradual process—one drink on the weeknights turns into two; two drinks on the weekends turns into four...you see where this is headed. I've never been a heavy drinker, and until we had our fifth child I think I could count the number of drinks I consumed on my fingers—I blame it all on my son. Before he was born, I would choose desserts over alcohol and then I'd be in a sugar coma before I was able to have a drink. After his birth, all bets were off and I *needed* that drink.

Before Christmas 2016, when things were pretty rough, and I probably should have taken medication to help deal with my depression, I thought I could handle it. I'd had some issues with depression before, and I guess I thought that since I'd walked this road before, I'd be able to find ways to cope with the tragedy and disappointment. Looking back, I can see I was actually using alcohol as a means of escape from what was going on, and I was also self-medicating.

This didn't work out well.

I know it sounds cliché, but when you're an artistic and creative person, this is pretty common. The burden of art and our weird little taste of celebrity, where we put our art and ourselves out there into the world, can cause some emotional weirdness, and I'll be the first to admit that maybe I wasn't cut out for it.

When I did my first extended fast in April 2017, it became *very* clear to me how dependent I was on my nightcap...or nightcaps. It was the way I slowed down my mind and relaxed. It was the way I could handle the stress of being a business owner, a mom, a wife, a farm owner, a friend, and a daughter...alcohol just helped me cope with it all. I don't think I'm alone in this, and I think it's pretty easy to do these days.

I'm not sure there's ever been a time in history when everyone seems to feel so heavy, so burdened. That's how I felt during that time. I was losing weight, but I'd never felt so heavy in my entire life. Some days it felt as if a 300-lb gorilla was sitting on my back and his brother was on my chest. It didn't feel good. Things eventually got better, but I still kept to my habit of relaxing with wine, usually after the kids went to bed. I've spoken to so many people who've said they often do the same thing. My mom didn't have a drink every night, nor did my grandmothers, but I think with the stressful culture we live in, regular drinking is more and more common.

Another unexpected side benefit of fasting was that I couldn't drink.

Or rather, I chose not to.

You want the straight truth? It was HARD AF.

For almost a year I'd routinely had at least one drink a night, and then when I did that first extended fast not only did I go without food or flavored drinks, I also didn't touch any alcohol. It really opened up my eyes to a few important things.

It forced me to come up with better ways to unwind and relax (more on that to come), and it made me realize I was so incredibly tense and stressed by the end of the day that it really wasn't healthy. It forced me to figure out other ways to cope with those stressful days, those days when I would say to Jack, "I *really* need a glass of wine." During those fasts, as I've said before, I felt more alert, I was more productive, I woke up with more energy because I was sleeping more deeply. I realized that some of this actually came from not only the fasting, but also from being totally sober during those times.

Even when I went back to having a glass of wine with dinner, even very dry red wine, I would sometimes get that "sugar slump" (which, BTW, I felt most often with white plates). My body just didn't like the effect of alcohol anymore.

Now I'm much more careful about what and when I drink, and also how much. I didn't realize before how easy it is for me to slip into these addictive patterns. I now know I have a super addictive personality—when I like something, I want more of it, and I usually don't stop until it becomes an issue. Jack would probably say it really wasn't that big of an issue, but whenever my health feels like it isn't headed in a positive direction, it feels that way to me. I was worried I was trading in one addiction for another, or maybe getting pretty close to it. Once I could see that drinking had the potential to hurt my health, my body, and my mind I decided I needed to be more careful about those choices.

My days look a lot different now than they did a year ago. I don't drink during the week anymore, and if I do I'm very careful to have lots of protein and fats with my meal so the effects of the alcohol on my body are lessened. Now, drinking is reserved for date nights or special occasions like publishing a new book.

In these books, I've always tried to be very candid with where I'm at, not just physically, but emotionally as well. I don't think everyone is as susceptible to this issue as I am, but I felt a responsibility to bring it to light. I think for many women who are on a weight-loss journey it's far too easy to replace food with other addictions.

I remember when I was working at the bariatric hospital; so many women would talk about having issues with drug and alcohol abuse, sexual addiction, and shopping addiction. When you have a personality that lends itself to addiction, it's important to be aware that some other addiction could very easily worm it's way into your life once you get a handle on one problem.

If you're one of my #wilderway sisters and you enjoy a glass of wine every night, I'm not at all trying to place any sort of judgment on you or your choices—I want to be very clear in that. I just needed to explain where I'm at with this.

Personally, I think I was at a point with alcohol where

I just couldn't get through a day without it, but now I don't want anything to have that sort of power over me. Not that I don't have hard days when I feel like I could really use a drink. Like today for example—all *six* of my kids are home from school because of an ice day, then a tree almost hit my car as I was driving one of my kids to piano, and then the UPS truck crashed after sliding down our driveway. So, yeah...I still have those days, but now I deal with them differently.

Tonight, I'll figure out other ways to relax and calm down after the kids are in bed. I might read or take a bath. Jack and I might "snuggle" and watch a comedy special. I might get *really* crazy and do a quick run, or walk around our property. The point is, I feel better knowing I have more control over my life.

Not turning to alcohol on a regular basis has also helped me gain control in other areas of my life. I became more aware of other places in my life where addiction was seeping in—more on that in further chapters.

If this is something you might be struggling with, please know you're not alone. I honestly think this might be a more common issue than most people think. So many of us struggle with addiction, trauma, and pain. It's okay to admit it and to actively work on it.

Our impulse is to want to be at the finish line in all things, all the time. Dude, I can't even tell you how badly I wish I was just "all good" with everything. Best mom—check; best wife—check; best writer—check; best at taking care of my body and mind—check and check! Well, my friends, that's just not where I am, not even on my best day! But I keep trying. I keep moving forward.

> We don't have to be perfect, mama! We just have to keep trying to be better than yesterday, and remember that being a champion means we keep going even when things aren't easy—*that's* winning.

Social Media Fasting

I KNOW YOU MIGHT HAVE BEEN EXPECTING THIS BOOK TO BE all about food, but it's really more about my health journey, and fasting from social media (FB, Instagram etc.) has been part of it. Over the past several years, when so much of my career has been spent online, I've seen my anxiety flare up and continue to get worse and worse. There are mornings when I've woken up legitimately fantasizing about the possibility of a sudden zombie apocalypse and all technology no longer exists. I would be freed of the shackle of my cell phone. Yes, I'd be running from zombies, but I would also have two hands free! I've had dreams about burying my cell phone and then singing "Amazing Grace" as I toss dirt on top of the tiny white coffin.

So last December, just before the holidays, I decided it was time to take a break from technology; that along with fasting from food, I would also do a social media (FACEBOOK) fast.

There is part of me that *hates* my phone as much as I love it. One thing I've learned about myself in this year of discovery/fasting/meditation is that I'm actually a solid intro-vert. I'm what the Enneagram calls a true romantic, a four—which means I *really* need solitude. I also know that with social media I never ever feel alone anymore. Again, this is both a good thing and a bad thing. But if I don't plan to have times to unplug, guess what happens to me? I slowly lose my mind. I do think my personality and lifestyle exacerbate this issue, but I know I'm not the only one.

The problems associated with being constantly connected are the things we tend to ignore until it gets out of hand. One thing I encourage, because of the changes I've experienced in my own life, is that you give yourself social media silence at the same time you give your body the healing benefits of abstain-ing from food. I can see all the eyeballs rolling as I say this, but we *need* rest from these things. It's too much—social media connectivity has truly become an epidemic in our society.

I'm seeing anxiety in our kids like never before, but then we're hooking our kids up to devices as never before, right? My oldest kids do 90 percent of their schoolwork on an iPad; they're looking at a screen almost the entire day, and you can't convince me this isn't damaging their developing brain. The increase in adolescent anxiety, restlessness, the inability to sleep at night, fear, and increased concern with appearances are, in my opinion, all related to overexposure to technology.

Even worse, this is a *curated* exposure. It isn't the real pic-ture, or the whole picture; it's the version of ourselves that we want people to see. I've always been pretty protective of the time my kids spent online, and none of my teenagers have any social media accounts.

But I didn't really make the strong connection between my own increase in restlessness and anxiety and online connectivity until things really came to a head with my stress levels. I took this as God showing me, in the clearest possible manner, that I was in need of a *serious* unplugging. Social media, the constant stream of input, the pressure to post and comment all day every day, the need to respond to EVERY email RIGHT AWAY—all this was contributing to a major anxiety crisis in my life; this anxiety pushed me to turn to wine in an attempt to escape the pressure and anxiety, but the more I drank, the more anxious I felt (see also the chapter on fasting from alcohol). This was a vicious cycle in my life, and I knew I had to find a way to break it.

How did I do it? I unplugged.

I've now made it a regular practice to take "unplugging" breaks—what some people call "going dark"—as part of my therapeutic fasting, so I can really, truly slow down and become more mindful, more in the moment. This does something for me akin to sitting on a beach on a tropical island. I can't entirely explain it, but my body, mind, and spirit all exhale as soon as I step away from technology, especially social media.

I know what you're saying: "WHAT IF I MISS SOMETHING?"

What if my cousin posts a birth announcement, and it's the cutest birth announcement ever? What if Target has a sale on Magnolia homeware? What if there are threats of nuclear war posted on Twitter and I'm the only person on the planet who didn't see it? Yes, these could be real concerns—I get it, there are things I sometimes worry about missing, too. But I really feel, deep in my soul, that there is *nothing* on the Internet more important than what's happening in your home, community, heart, body, mind, and soul. Literally *nothing*. If by some chance something literally life changing is happening, my guess is someone will let you in on it.

I can honestly say my mental wellness, restfulness, and sense of peace is deeply connected to my reduced social media intake; I have added literal hours to my day simply by cutting out or least significantly cutting down on time spent on electronic devices. I now count the minutes I spend on social media like I count glasses of wine.

I have even gone so far as to completely turn off my phone and put it in a drawer in my bedroom. I do this especially on Sundays and during family time, so I don't feel the pressure or temptation to even look at it. If you have your phone on and nearby, you WILL open it up and look at it. Putting it completely away removes that impulse from you, which I've found to be another huge stress reliever.

> Dull the sparkle: in iPhones—and probably Androids, but I'm not sure as I've never owned one—you can go into your display settings and set your phone to grayscale, so everything is in black, white, and gray. Less color and shine equals less draw toward those little red notifications, and less temptation to endlessly scroll.

Social media is absolutely fine in moderation, but when it consumes you and makes your life harder, more complicated, and starts to steal your joy...it's time to change some things. Right?

> To really simplify your digital life, I have two suggestions. First, delete unnecessary or unused apps—they just take up space on your phone and real estate on your screen. Second, unsubscribe from those junk email lists; all they do is clutter up your inbox and tempt you with garbage you don't need!

Now, if you want to get some super bonus #wilderway points, I'm going to suggest you try a social media fast during your eight-week challenge. Just see how you feel. Do you sleep better? Are you resting more deeply? Are you less anxious?

Try it and tag me: #wilderwaysocialmediafasting.

That was a trick! Don't do it! Stay off social media! It's a trap!

For real though, just try to cut back on social media a bit while you are food fasting, and JOURNAL about it! You'll have so much extra time that you could write a book, or you'll have so much energy from being well rested that you could run a half marathon, or you'll be inspired to clean every closet in your house. It could happen!

Fasting from Yes

(AKA A BEAUTIFUL SEASON OF "NO'S")

It's funny to admit this, but people often ask me how I can write so many books and be a mom to six kids and have a farm and still shower occasionally, but the honest answer is I really don't know myself. Jack is a great help and I couldn't do it without him as my partner—THANK YOU, JESUS! Honestly, I'm very choosy with my time management, and this past year it has become abundantly clear to me that I need to be even *more* choosy. Just because something is "happening" doesn't mean it's something that I *need* to do.

I'm a very choosy mom: we don't do playdates or birthday parties or many nights away from home after school. We pick our extracurricular activities carefully. I'm not a classroom mom. I say no to most events. My kids get asked to participate in the school play, but it would mean we would never eat dinner together or finish our homework—so we say NO. We end up saying no much more often than we say yes.

There was a point when all we said was "YES, YES,

YES"...and then I hit a wall and we entered a season of NO. This has been *so* liberating and joyful, my friends.

There's freedom in saying NO. Again, I know it seems like my family is missing out on a lot of amazing things, but what I've learned from this is that when we say no, there's often a secret YES God is waiting to bless us with.

Nothing clarified this for me as much as when we slowed down our travel schedule. I had a pit in my stomach when we decided to cut back, worried that it was a career ender. How would I stay relevant? How would people remember me? How could I get the word out about new books? How would I get over missing the hugs, the love, and the people that made me feel like I was "something"?

Guys, this was also HARD AF.

The love from my readers was like a drug, and the first time I had to say no to an event I basically had a feeling like "well, this is over now. Pack it all up. I'm done." I cried real tears. But what I heard from God during this time was that this wasn't all about me. My readers didn't love *me*, they loved my books—and when I thought about it that was really what I wanted to be remembered for. The connection my readers had with me was all through my words and my characters. Being away from my office so frequently was hurting my writing. The recovery time from travel is no joke; it can take DAYS for me to get over a weekend event.

When I'm dead and gone who do I want to remember me? My kids.

What do I want my readers to remember? My characters,

my stories.

Those are my legacies, plain and simple.

When we began reducing our time away, there were times I would be on Facebook looking at the photos of my author friends, bloggers, and readers who had become friends, and I would be so sad I was missing out. Let me tell you, each and every time this sort of thing happened life would hug me in a serious way. Each and every time I made that difficult choice and said no, something at home would affirm that I had made the right choice.

The pressure on women—especially mothers—is CRAZY. Let's be honest, being a mom has always been hard, but many of us are now working and trying desperately to balance all the things Pinterest is telling us we need to do, and we're frantically hustling from one commitment to the next.

We don't need another pedicure or lunch date; what we need is some quietude, the kind of quiet you have to fight for, the kind you have to carve out for yourself. Many of us have no idea how to achieve that kind of quiet.

Yoga? Hot yoga? A Jesuit retreat?

Most of us could get a good start on it by just saying no as much as we say yes. We want to be liked. We want to be YES-people, while so many of us are screaming inside to say no.

Well, I want to inspire the no-person inside you. Say no to the school PTO so you can sit with yourself and God for five minutes. Say no to making the sugar-free unicorn cake for the cake walk so you can write in a prayer journal for your family—not just quick prayer in your head, but rather give yourself a full ten minutes. I know this might seem impossible seeing as you haven't done laundry since, like, Lent, but I promise you those ten minutes will be worth it.

And listen, if I'm not singing your song right now, you're probably a way more balanced person than I am. I'm finding the longer I'm on this earth—and the longer I'm on this earth as a mother—that mom guilt and mom regret is a real thing. We don't get this time back, and it flies by all too quickly. If we can become intentional about the quality of our life, and allow ourselves to be less influenced by the stuff that really isn't important in the long run, I think we'll all be happier mamas.

Make a list right now of the things in your life that are most demanding. My guess is there are many things you do each day that don't even make the list. Cross those puppies off *right now* and write "NO!" beside each and every one.

I have a list of about ten things right now that get my full-time commitment and attention, and everything else is a no. The cool thing is that this has freed me up to say YES to things that I wouldn't have imagined.

Saying no leads to a secret yes, and the secret yes is *magical.*

So I didn't go to that awesome event in New York last summer, but I *did* get to do four-day work weeks for an entire month and went to see an artsy matinee show with my husband every Friday of each of those weeks. That was an awesome secret my secret yes life gave me, and which I continue to be inspired and refreshed by.

Just for fun, and just to get you thinking, below is my Top Ten List of things to say no to.

TEN THINGS TO SAY NO TO RIGHT NOW:

1. Palazzo pants
2. Foods with ingredients you can't pronounce
3. Movies with Nicholas Cage as the lead
4. Lip injections and/or butt implants
5. Self-hatred
6. Vacations to northern Michigan in January (unless you love the feel of a balmy -15 on your face)
7. Coca-Cola
8. Mom jeans
9. Sugar
10. Global warming

A list of things to say YES to:

TEN THINGS TO SAY YES TO RIGHT NOW:

1. Dry shampoo
2. Marcona almonds with oil and salt
3. Movies with Hugh Jackman
4. Zevia soda or LaCroix
5. Rose gold anything!
6. Vacations to northern Michigan in August (BEAUTI-FUL! I suggest beaches and a wine tour)

7. A good book
8. Bacon
9. Red shoes
10. #wilderway chocolate cake for breakfast

Fasting from All the Things

SIMPLIFY

ALMOST AS A JOKE IN AN EARLIER CHAPTER I MENTIONED how having all this extra time and energy on your hands will give you the motivation to clean out your closets and organize your kitchen.

Okay...I really wasn't totally joking about that. When you do have extra energy I think it's only natural that your body and mind will want to spend it on productive things like work, organization, and running. For me, I had so many years of chronic fatigue that once I started to feel better and had so much more energy, running came as a natural response. I just wanted to get out and get moving. If you had told me when I weighed 300-plus pounds that my body and mind would respond this way to losing weight, I would have laughed at you.

The body and mind do some odd things.

Another thing that has happened as a response to having

extra energy is wanting to become more organized and get rid of the things that I think literally "weighed me down." I realized that we have so much crap we never use, junk we don't need, clothes we probably won't wear again, soap under the sink that has been there for years. I'm really not a hoarder, I promise, but this is just life in the busy lane when you have a bunch of kids, a career, and feel overextended 80 percent of the time.

> Random true fact for you: the average American household contains 300,000 individual items. I'm going to write that number out, as emphasis: THREE HUNDRED THOUSAND items. That, my friends, is a lot of stuff. Things just sort of accumulate, don't they? Why did I have five ladles when I only use one? This is the type of thing that started occurring to me.

Clothes have always been a really big issue for me. When I was a kid my mom would take me to Sears into the plus-sized kids' section, which I'm pretty sure they called "hefty" or something equally horrible, and we would just buy whatever we could find that would fit; I didn't have options, and there was no such thing as fashion. I also had huge feet as a child, and again, whereas my sister had about fourteen different types of shoes to choose from, I was lucky if we could find a single pair that would fit which didn't totally look like boy shoes. Sometimes I cried because the shoes were so ugly.

I also remember my mom calling stores in New York City trying to find me shoes that weren't all black with Velcro, because there was a period of time when that was literally all we could find for me in the metro Detroit area. Thank goodness the Internet came along and made finding things easier. Right, Mom?

This clothing thing has continued to plague me. Even when I got down to a size where I could fit into Lane Bryant clothing and everything wasn't black pants and floral tops, I still usually just bought whatever fit the best. I wasn't exactly able to throw fashion into the equation when I was just trying to stuff my booty and legs into any pants that didn't come from a catalogue. When I reached a point where I could wear "normal" sizes, I started to feel a sort of high when things with an "M" on the tag fit over my boobs, and it became *so* difficult to say no to new clothes. And listen, you all know I'm thrifty so I'm not talking about designer brands here, I'm talking about walking into Target or Gap and having a 20 percent off coupon and everything not only fits but looks decent on you. It's a trap!

During this part of the journey, my closets started to burst a bit. I'm not even sure when I thought I was going to wear ten black shirts of various length. Hey, I like black, but one thing I realized was I always gravitate to the same things over and over again, and all the other stuff in the closet just gets in the way of finding the things I like.

So, since I'm talking to you about these kinds of changes, I want to lay this out for you too: don't let your stuff weigh you down. The things you have around you should be your best things. The things that make you smile. The things you go to time and again. The things that make you *you*.

Don't have so many *things* that the important stuff can't be seen. Don't save your favorite things for a day that never comes; that's another thing I always did! I don't even know why. I guess I felt I always had to save the best things for "a special occasion." Jack and I would go to a signing event and I would come home never having worn the outfit I liked best. I can't even really explain to you why, other than I just always want to save the best. I hold on to the dress for a perfect occasion that never comes, or I'll save the good plates for a dinner party that never happens, the statement necklace for a gala I'm never invited to, a running outfit for the perfect race, heels for a red carpet I'll never walk.

This is NOT LIVING! This is saving things for an imaginary future day you think will be perfect—that day is *today*. We tend to forget those things are even there because we've covered them up. They're sitting at the very back of the closet waiting for...what? Waiting for us to feel worthy to wear them? I'm not sure.

During this season of feasting and fasting, I've looked into my closet, asked myself a few questions, and come to a few conclusions:

- Which clothes feel good, look good, and make me feel and look like an authentic me, even if that doesn't look like everyone else?

- Which things are my favorites? Put those things front and center, and if you really love something, WEAR IT! Those red shoes that you love but are saving for the perfect event? Put those puppies on *today*! Today is just as good as any to feel great! I really think too many of us are saving up for perfect Instagrammable moments, and we miss out on the joys of normal, beautiful days.

- Give away, gift away, donate, and toss! If there's something you have that you don't use, I promise you there's someone out there in this world who would probably love to have it and use it. One of our local churches has a community garage sale where we put out anything we think might be of value. People are free to just come and take what they need. I'm sure you can find something similar in your community. See if there's a women's shelter nearby—they can always use clothing. You can even resale or do a trade day with friends. Invite friends over for coffee and have them bring jewelry, clothes, shoes, or other items they want to trade. That scarf might not be your thing anymore, but it might be exactly what your friend is looking for.

- Tidy Tuesday: Every Tuesday, my family goes through a particular area of our home, sorting through belongings, and we find things we no longer love, no longer use, or no longer need, and we get rid of it. If it's garbage, we toss it, if it's reusable we either sell it or donate it. For us, this is a way of simplifying our lives by shedding unneeded items. This has the added bonus of helping us find and focus in on those items which we really truly love the best and use the most. Which leads me to the next tip…

- If you haven't used something in the past six to twelve months, you won't ever use it again, I promise. I come from grandparents who remembered the depression—they kept scraps of tinfoil if they thought they could use it again. In all honesty, if we don't use something on a regular basis, it really isn't doing anything for us. Clutter and things and possessions can become burdens.

There are some awesome apps out there that'll even help you figure out what clothes you wear the most.

- Listen, I'm not asking you to go throw away everything you own, I'm just asking you to try to sort through one closet, or one drawer in your pantry, and see if you don't feel better. I can all but guarantee you will. There's freedom in this. You can do it!

Fasting from Negativity

I CAN'T THINK OF A TIME IN MY LIFE WHEN I DIDN'T daydream about being someone else, anyone else—my life was just too hard. There were too many judgmental eyes always focused on me. There was so much self-loathing and shame and anger and just plain yuckiness. I hid it well most of the time. Most of my life was spent being the funny fat girl, and I did it pretty well. I kept the shame close to my heart, never really letting all of the dark parts inside me spill out into the open. And when I did get really down and depressed, there was always food to comfort me. I repeated this cycle for most of my life.

I remember losing some weight during my senior year of high school, only to gain it all back during my freshman year of college. Senior year was full of joy for me—I felt like I made it: I hadn't become a teen mom, I had decent grades,

I'd been accepted into all of the schools I had applied to, with scholarships to boot. Things were looking pretty good! Then all heck broke loose my freshman year of college and I resorted to the old patterns. I ate myself back to calmness. This just created more self-loathing that led to more eating. Again and again I would get on this same, destructive train. I *never* felt okay. I *never* wanted to be who I was. The grass is always greener, right? It's especially true with your body.

Still, to this day, I look at people on weight-loss journeys on social media and I think, "Gosh, their loss is so much more dramatic than mine. She doesn't have as much hanging skin. She isn't as old. Why couldn't I lose the weight sooner? Why will I never be able to see my body in its actual prime condition without all the wrinkles, and skin, and imperfections?" This is really what does go through my head almost every day. Jasinda—pity party for one.

It's so much easier for me to think this way than to think of all of the things that are going right. I lose sight of the good things, the ways my body has changed for the positive. There's just something constantly drawing me back to the negative. I know I'm not the only one out there who has this issue. SO many women have confided in me that *this* is the struggle which so often keeps them in the loop of seeking comfort in food, keeping them on the cycle of negative reinforcement and negative self-talk.

Here's what I've learned.

I think women who have struggled with their weight their whole lives often fantasize about a different life, or a different body. We think about how our lives will suddenly just be "prime." We'll no longer struggle with the demons. We'll look perfect in the swimsuit, we'll accomplish things we never have before; we'll be at the top of the mountain.

Yes, some things do become "easier" when you lose weight. There are things I can do now that I couldn't do at 430 lbs, but I was still living the same life back then. There were still good things. Even at my current weight I still struggle, I still lack confidence in my body; I still flounder with my emotions and strive to cope with them in a healthy way. Life is full of challenges, and this particular journey is just one of many for me.

What I've found to be the most important factor in how we enjoy life is what we focus on. In my experience, this is a choice. In my house we have a big sign over the door that reads JOY. I probably say "choose joy" to my kids at least a half a dozen times each and every day, and I say it to myself. I have to keep saying it, and I have to say it out loud because if I don't my mind ends right back up in negativity. From the outside, my life looks pretty darn good. Beautiful farm, healthy for the first time in my life, six healthy children, a sexy husband... but so often my mind is lost in the "worst possible scenario" wilderness.

I look in the mirror and see all the things that are wrong with me—I made too many mistakes; I ruined a relationship; I'm never enough and never will be. Once I've started the downward spiral I start to think about cupcakes... yes, cupcakes will make this all better. This is a tale as old as time, for me. Even as I sit here thinking about it, I feel weak. This is why I have purposely set up what I call my "safety net." I always have some sort of "healthier chocolate" nearby I can dip into natural peanut butter. I keep some Dr. John's caramels in my pantry or desk drawer. I have Halo Top ice cream in the freezer, and I have Skinny popcorn in the cupboard. Not because I need it every day, but I want to have some better choices around if I feel myself getting triggered. This is one of the best ways I can love myself. When I find myself in that place, I go to something that isn't harmful to my body. This safety net has saved me more times than I can say.

As I've said previously, the other thing that has really made a huge change in my mindset is taking time every day to focus on the good. What is going right? What are my blessings today? What do I like about my body? What can I affirm for myself that might outweigh my fears? I've learned that being proactive against a negative mindset has very literally changed my life. I've even found that doing this with my kids has made a pretty big difference in their outlooks.

> This might look a bit different for you and that's okay. Through my personal coaching sessions I've found talking about the good things really needs to be fluid. Sometimes you need to list a few affirmations, and then there are days it's important to list every single blessing we can think of.

I really recommend that you set yourself up with a Blessing Journal. For me, writing in a journal was a big step, and it actually felt better to get this stuff all out, and have a running documentation of where I've been and where I hope to go. It's a testimony of all the good things. Those really bad days, the ones where I just can't see the light, are the days when I go back to the start of my journal and reread all of my blessings.

This feels so good, friends. It creates a buffer around that particular moment or day, and makes it so much easier to see how good we really have it. I've made a habit of writing out a quick list of blessings every morning. You can include anything on this list, and you don't have to spend a ton of time thinking about it. Give yourself about five minutes or less. If you forget to do it in the morning, and then remember a few hours later, pull out your smartphone and make a quick note. You can always transfer it over into your journal later. Some days I just meditate on those things for a few minutes. How can you not feel good when you think about the good things?

A LIST OF MY GOOD THINGS

- My warm bed
- Coffee
- Being able to do what I love
- Books and time to read them
- My comfy chair

There are days when five are enough and I think about those things and really feel my heart well up with thanks.

Other days I will sit and write twenty. One day I decided that I needed to list a solid fifty things that stood out as blessings in my life. That was the day I had to get out of the trap my mind was leading me into.

I *am* enough, and I *have* enough.

My cup is half-full.

Good things are all around me.

I know it sounds trite, but this simple act can make such a *huge* difference when you make it a practice. I promise you, spending those moments where you meditate on the good things will stick with you. It will tuck into a corner of your brain and sit there and pop out when you least expect it.

It's funny, because so often my chair makes it to my list. It's a turquoise chair that feels like it was molded and made just for my body. It's such a good thing that probably once a week it will be listed in my blessings—I love it that much! When I'm struggling, I can just think of my chair and it brings a smile to my face. Maybe you have some special place that brings those good feelings to you—put yourself there in your mind even if you can't physically be there. Your physical happy place will become your mental happy place.

When I'm done with my blessings, I write out my affirmations. Again, I know this may sound silly, but I truly believe that what we put out into the universe is really important. I believe in intention, in the power of words, written and spoken.

There are days when I feel as if all of my affirmations need to be about my body:

- I have beautiful, strong legs.
- I am healthy.
- I am wise and make good decisions.
- I can run.
- I am whole and worthy.

There are other days when my affirmations need to be about my career or my children, and there are days when my affirmations are all over the place, about all sorts of things:

- I have a good, strong marriage to my best friend. We grow closer to each other every single day.
- The food I put into my body brings me closer to good health.
- My children are healthy and safe.
- I am whole and my body is beautiful.
- I sleep well and wake up each day feeling refreshed and well rested.

I had a day recently when I wrote several pages of affirmations because I really needed to get them out. I went through each section of my life where negative thoughts creep in—my husband, my kids, my career, my body, my finances, my faith. Once I have those things down in my journal, I go back to them when I need to refocus. Sometimes writing them into my journal is enough, and other days I have to actually say them out loud to myself.

Over the past year of doing this very purposefully and intentionally, negativity has had less and less of a hold on me. I'm still a work in progress, and there are days when I feel down, but journaling has really helped me see my life, my day, my body, my relationships, and this journey as a blessing rather than a curse.

A few years ago I would have had a hard time if someone even tried to tell me I was pretty—yes, I would've probably flinched—now I am able to feel more comfortable with compliments about my body. When my mind starts to go over the things I'm lacking in regards to my body, I am able to pull up a list of all of the things that I like about myself, including all of my mental and physical strengths.

Each one of my self-help books represents a season for me in my wellness journey. When I look back I see the places where I had to take a turn, or go down a different path. I can't believe how much of this has been mental for me. The body part was actually a bit easier for me than the mental process. I wasn't prepared for all of those ghosts in my closet, for all of the emotion and the doubts and the negativity that crept up to the surface of my psyche.

I've changed. I'm not the same Jasinda I was a year ago—well, I am in some ways, but I'm also not. The core parts, which make me, *me* are all still there, but hopefully now I'm Jasinda 2.0.

This journey has really opened up new things for me, some of which I'm not sure I would have ever understood had I not made these physical changes. Once the body undergoes this sort of drastic change, I believe it's only natural for the mind to follow.

I think as women we often use food as a way to quiet our

minds and avoid the things that are troubling us by causing a "fullness" inside of us, which then turns off that nagging voice in our minds. Once I didn't have food to fill that hole, these mental issues really came forward and became louder. As I was shedding weight I was also peeling back layers. Journaling really helped me work through those layers.

I also found it helpful to talk to someone about how I was feeling, so I went to a counselor. I needed someone who wasn't my husband to help me process the changes I was going through, and to work out some of the body image issues I was still feeling. It was very important that I discuss what my ideal body would be versus what my body is now, and not only embrace my new body but love it.

I'm not sure this is something we discuss enough when we talk about weight loss and body image, and it should be, so I'm saying it here. If you need to talk to someone during this journey, DO IT! It doesn't make you weak—I believe it actually makes you stronger.

There is no shame in seeking counsel or therapy.

So many of us are victims of abuse, and when you can no longer stifle that abuse with food you need to figure out different ways to work through your emotions, fears, and sorrows.

This is okay. This is good.

Take care of you: you'll never, ever regret the work you spend on yourself.

Below are some ideas to get started on writing your own journal:

JOURNAL STARTERS:

- What are you thankful for today? Try to list at least five things.
- What is going right today?
- What is good about your body today?
- What positive things are you proud of?
- What brings you the greatest joy?
- What do you like about yourself?
- What unexpected blessings have you witnessed?
- What was the best part of your day and the most challenging part of your day?
- How has the world shown you that you are loved today?
- How does the food you're eating make you feel?
- What foods make you feel the best?
- When was the time when you felt best about your body?
- In what ways have you been successful in this new lifestyle?
- If love could speak, what would it say to you today?
- How do you feel when you're fasting? How does your body feel? How does your mind feel?
- How do you feel about your body today?
- How do you *want* to feel about your body?
- List five to ten things you're grateful for.
- How have you grown or changed on your journey this week?

- I am proud of myself because _____.
- Dear past me…
- Dear future me…
- What should be my reward for reaching my goals?

Giving Yourself Grace

I'M WRITING THIS CHAPTER MOSTLY FOR MYSELF. I'M NOT sure it will resonate with everyone, but it's something that I feel needs to be said because I needed to hear it, and so I want to share it with you.

In a sermon recently, my pastor said that grace is unmerited kindness.

Grace is something I've talked about a lot in these books. For most people, grace is reserved for church, or talking about spirituality, but I want to chat for a moment about what it really means when I tell you to give yourself grace on this journey.

For most of my life I've felt intense shame about the way my body looked. This is a deeply rooted shame that is still, after thirty-eight years, very difficult for me to talk about, and I guess maybe that's why I am writing about it. I can't even remember a time in my life when I didn't feel shame, and that shame not only shaped me as a person, but it also controlled me. I always felt bad for my parents, my sister, my friends, or anyone who had to deal with me. My body often held me and others back from things in life. There were concerts we couldn't attend, cars we couldn't fit in, times when people yelled horrible things that my friends and family felt they had to defend against. It really wasn't fun most days having to deal with my body. It's something most people wouldn't understand unless they've lived it.

Life at 430 lbs is mostly a struggle, mostly hard, and mostly painful.

I never gave myself grace. I would try and fail, try and fail, and try and fail again, and every single time I failed I felt worse about myself. I never gave myself grace, and that would just add to the shame, and then the next time I failed I would think, "Well, you're just never going to do this. You don't deserve this. You are a horrible person with no willpower and you won't ever overcome this."

As I've said before, the mind is a very powerful thing and I think that's why it's been so hard to really know and understand grace.

What we think about ourselves becomes our truth.

Grace seems like it should be so easy, especially with ourselves, but I've found in my own journey, as well as through coaching other ladies, that grace is often the hardest thing to give ourselves. Why is it so hard to give ourselves unmerited kindness along this journey? I think at the core it has to do with shame.

So many of are burdened with shame because of our choices, or the state of our bodies, that we can't be kind to ourselves anymore. All we feel is anger, hatred, and disgust. Trust me, I understand—I've been there. Heck, some days I'm *still* there. But what I know about grace is that it's there for everyone, if we choose it. It's right there in front of us, a gift we can either accept or refuse.

Accepting grace can mean the difference between success and failure. I've seen this over and over again, and never as clearly as with one of the women I have been coaching. She's going through a pretty rough stretch of life at the moment. She's been through health crisis after health crisis, and she's lost and gained weight so many times she's lost count. Each time she gained it back, she felt worse and worse about herself. She and her husband are navigating their way through financial setbacks, and they have a sick family member they're trying to care for. Honestly, it seems like it couldn't get any worse for them.

When we first started our sessions, she was so hard on herself that it would pain me to listen to her. I don't think she even believed she deserved good things anymore. My only hope was that she had set up these sessions with me, so she must have had *some* hope that things would get better. She beat herself up verbally and only spoke about all the things she was doing wrong even when she did so many things right. The negative voices in her head were always talking so loudly that she couldn't drown them out.

We started with small exercises—I made her say *one* positive thing about herself, *one* thing she was doing right, and then we would figure out one affirmation she would work on throughout the week. I told her she needed to not only continue to write this affirmation out, but also speak it to herself out loud. Sometimes we need to say these things—I mean really verbally say them out loud. We have to speak positively to ourselves even if we don't feel that way yet.

Our next two sessions were her trying to tell me how she couldn't do this. It was basically ten minutes of her explaining why she couldn't and twenty minutes of me explaining why she could and should and would. Every single session ended with me talking about how she needed to give herself some grace. One bad choice or one bad day wouldn't ruin her progress—this isn't an all-or-nothing plan, your health isn't riding on one bad decision. As I've said over and over again, just as all the not-so-great choices brought you to the health issues you have today, all the good choices can lead you to good health.

This is cumulative, and these good choices add up!

Session four I could tell that something was changing in her. She was kinder when she was talking about herself. She wasn't perfect with her eating plan or journaling, but she wasn't beating herself up like she had been in previous sessions. It was almost like talking to a totally different person.

I told her how proud I was of her and we mapped out her eating and journaling plan for the next week. When I talked with her in the next session she was almost glowing, and nearly crying. She had been in a stall for months before this, I think mostly from lack of sleep and stress, but she had finally broken the stall and was so upbeat and positive about the changes she was making.

I asked her to talk about herself and what she thought she

had done well for that week, and for twenty minutes she went on and on about what she had cooked, how she had planned for her travel commitment, and how she had been successful with the food she had brought with her. She was so excited about her progress, and she was finally seeing herself in a better light. Her outlook was so drastically different from when we first started our sessions that I thought, "This isn't even the same woman!"

It was amazing what giving herself some grace had done for her! When we ended that session I actually burst into tears of joy. Just as it had pained me to hear her talk about herself weeks ago, now it was bringing me joy to hear her talk about how good she felt and how proud she was of herself.

Amazing grace!

None of this was because of something *I* did. This was something she had to do for herself; she put in a lot of very hard work so she could look at herself, her life, and her situation in a different way. The thing is, not many of those outside factors had changed. She was still under a great deal of stress, but she was taking care of herself with kindness, and that made it possible for her to better manage what life was throwing at her.

How often do we think that once our situation changes, once we get this one thing in order, once we put out this fire, get to this size, or get this thing done, *then* we'll start taking care of ourselves, *then* we'll start really living life, *then* everything will be good. Today isn't the day, but tomorrow will be. I just need to get to a certain point first, and *then* I'll love who I am, and be loving toward myself.

You deserve that right now, *today*. I know for most of us it just doesn't feel that way. There are too many parts not to love, too many bad things we've done, too much going wrong, too much stress. I understand. I'm fighting the same thing every single day of my life.

> A very wise person once told me it's those things we hate about ourselves the most that really need the most love because that's how we heal.

Instead of living with the shame of mistakes, shortcomings, scars, or regret we can choose grace. We can choose to live in a way that shows love to ourselves through our words, actions, and thoughts, regardless if we think it's merited or not. Giving yourself grace is one of the most beautiful and difficult things you can do. But friends, *please* do it.

You are worthy.

You are good enough.

Please accept the gift, and when you stumble, remind yourself that you always have the chance to try again.

As Jack tells my kids, you miss 100 percent of the shots you don't take.

Keep trying and keep giving yourself GRACE!

You can do it!

Update: Body Dysmorphia

I WANT TO TOUCH ON THE SUBJECT OF BODY DYSMORPHIA, since I did bring up my struggle with it in the previous book. Am I still working on this? Yes. My biggest issue is still just feeling big. I still worry whether I can fit into a chair, or if I'll be told I'm too big for a roller coaster ride, or if I'll still go into a dressing room with clothes WAY too big for me.

Often, when I see myself in the mirror or in photos, I don't recognize myself at all. The really weird part of it is that I don't recognize the girl I am, but I'm also not who I used to be, or who I thought I would be. I still harbor the fantasy that one day I will be a vision of perfect health, and that makes truly seeing myself now a bit more difficult.

When I was in high school I would spend hours day-dreaming about what I would look like if I ever lost all my weight and no longer had health problems. This was something I obsessed over because, at the time, my singing was getting noticed and there were whispers about my being able to "make it big" if I could lose the weight. I would create visions of singing on a big stage, glowing, both muscular and slender, in a beautiful gown, my face bursting with happiness because of the love coming from my fans. Yes, I was a teenager, and teenagers all have "success fantasies," but this was a hard dream to pull off when I was sitting there at 350 lbs eating my superman ice cream.

A fantasy like this is both good and bad; it was bad because it was so unrealistic, but it was also good because it gave me something to look forward to, something to hope for. Now, after years and years of struggling with my body image fantasies, versus what I actually looked like, I understand why this body dysmorphia issue is still going on. I've spent thirty-five years with my body looking one way, and thirty-five years imagining how my body would look one day. Both these images are stuck in my mind...but I'm currently neither of those things. What I am is something totally different, totally new, but still good...just different. It'll take some time for me to really "get" this new me. And sometimes it does feel like this whole process is going *so* slowly.

Why can't I just get over this? Why can't I just be fine? Why is making peace with my body, and this journey, so dang hard? Why can't I just look in the mirror and see, finally, for *once* who I am and be okay and proud of that person?

I wish I had a better answer for you other than this stuff just takes a lot of time and a lot of work. I told my doctor it's a lot like a person who's been blind their whole life and are finally able to see, or someone who suddenly loses a limb, or a deaf person who is finally able to hear? It's both physical and mental, so it takes time for your brain to process the changes, to truly, deeply understand that you aren't who you once were physically, and your body has to adjust to these changes.

It's okay if you're at this place in your journey. It's okay if it takes time for you to really see and feel your body for what it is now. There's no special, magical way to rush this process. There's no way to make it happen any sooner. I wish there was, trust me. For me, this has been one of the most difficult parts of the journey, because it's tied into not only loving myself, but also to appreciating the body I have now. It's tied into taking care of my body, seeing it for all of the wonderful things it has already accomplished, and recognizing all of the wonderful things it has yet to do!

Jack is constantly telling me I can do stuff I just assume I can't. I can't lift this, I can't jump that, I can't run that far, I can't get into a canoe—have I ever told the story about the time I tipped a paddle boat with my friends in it just trying to get in? Living the way I did my entire life, my instinct is just to think my body won't be able to do something. There's a whole list of things I just imagined I would never be able to do my entire life. If you've never been 300 or 400 lbs it might be hard to imagine, but I never thought I would ski, I never thought I would be able to mountain climb, run or swim a great distance, ride in one of those really tiny sports cars. I know it sounds crazy, but I would honestly sit and think about the things I would miss out on in life because of my size. It was something that had just become part of my life, and now that little voice in my head is still there and doesn't want to leave. The eviction notice has been delivered and I'm happy to say I'm finally starting to believe that, physically, there is nothing that I can't do.

Boom!

Karri has also been so helpful in this area, especially when it comes to seeing what I can wear and what's just too darn big. I know I talked about this in the previous book, but you would think over a year later I'd have gotten with the program on this. Currently I usually wear a size medium. I can't even tell you how hard Karri had to push to even get me to admit that my size large clothing was getting too big. I was literally fighting with her almost daily about how my clothes were not falling off me. The Stitch Fix box I got quarterly would come and she would tell me everything was too big. Unconvinced, she would grab my app and look at the sizes I had ordered and then tell me all of those sizes were at least two sizes too big. Again, I don't know why this is such a weird mental hang-up for me, but I'm really trying to get over it.

When I think about my comfy 6X Michigan State Football hoodie I wore all through college I guess it might make sense now that picking up a size medium in anything still feels a bit unnatural. I know this might sound like a really weird problem to have, but I'm sure some of you out there might relate to it.

Every day I fight to embrace the size, shape, state, and composition of my body. Here are a few things I've done which have really helped me get comfortable with my body, both physically and mentally:

- I take photos of myself. Different angles, naked, clothed, all done up, and looking like I just woke up. I look at those photos and make sure positive things run through my head. I force it a bit if I have to, but I really look for the good things in each photo and praise my body for what it is.

- YOGA, YOGA, YOGA! Have I mentioned yoga, yet? I know I sound like a broken record, but yoga has basically saved my life. The type of yoga I practice now is specifically meant to heal the body. Yoga helps you feel things, meditate, get quiet, and be still. When I practice yoga I really get a better understanding of my body and I'm at peace with it. If you've never done any yoga before and you're at any stage in this journey, I highly recommend you try to find a class in your area. My class is for all levels and I'm pretty sure the oldest person in my class is almost ninety, so anyone can do this. It's great for your body, mind, and soul! More on this in the next chapter.

- Meditation: If you're too scared to get out there and try a class, I would recommend trying a positive meditation app or some other audio that will help you get into a space where you can focus on good, positive things about your body and how you look and feel. I've never really understood how big the mental component is to this journey until recently, but it truly is key. If you aren't in a good place with yourself mentally, the physical journey will just be that much harder. Two apps I recommend for this: Calm, and 10% Happier.

- Look in the mirror and say good things about yourself. I know, I know, there's no way you can do that—it's weird and awkward and strange. But do you know how many negative things you say about yourself without even noticing it? It takes seven positive things to counter just one negative. I want you to try and notice today when you have a negative thought about yourself; I bet it'll be more often than you think. Whenever I go to the bathroom—which is a lot since I drink coffee and water all day long—I stop, look in the mirror, and say at least one positive thing about myself. Yes, this is on top of my daily affirmations. There's no limit on the good things you can think about yourself, or the positive ways you can look at yourself. We are surrounded by negativity, so take time to really look at yourself and see all the good things. Say them out loud; say them twice. I want to hear you all the way over here in Michigan! Bonus points if you sing them to yourself like a Disney princess and then do a self-hug. Just kidding. Well… mostly kidding.

- Only wear what makes you feel good. Again, this is something that might also seem silly, but stop wearing clothes that don't fit or don't make you feel good. Wear the black dress, wear the black heels, buy jeans that aren't falling off you, stop wearing yoga pants every single day. Yes there's a time and a place for comfy clothes, but it's so hard for many of us to embrace the fact that we can wear things we had on the "I'll never wear these" list for so long. Find a few items that really make you feel good and WEAR THEM. Get rid of the stuff that doesn't flatter you. Enlist a friend if you need help or advice with this. You can go to a second-hand or consignment store, or use the Mercari app to trade stuff that's too big and save money. I also suggest getting some sexy red heels—it's impossible not to feel sexy in some red pumps ladies. I promise!

Self-Care 101

I'M EMBARRASSED TO SAY I REALLY HAVEN'T DONE MUCH positive self-care until very recently. And when you have five or six kids, even getting dressed or showered can feel like self-care if you spend more than twenty minutes doing those things.

However, if I'm being honest, I guess I never felt as if I deserved it; and that's the 100 percent truth. For most of my adult life my self-care looked like this: I rewarded myself with food. Yes, food was my reward and, on occasion, maybe I'd treat myself to a new purse, or some new makeup. I would also get a pedicure every so often, and that felt like some serious indulgence, too. But if I was really good, I got myself a cupcake. This reward system always made me feel better momentarily, and it gave me the illusion of self-care.

Of course when you're fasting you literally can't reward yourself with food. It is simply not an option. So...what do you do?

Once I didn't have my usual food rewards I had to

reevaluate what self-care really was, and what it should actually look like. I know this might sound lame and silly, but this is something I hadn't really thought much about, because I'd been using the same food reward system for myself since childhood. I'm being really honest here, because my guess is that if I did this, maybe some of you did it too. I had been on a crazy rollercoaster of rewarding and punishing myself for decades, and I had to figure out a new way to take care of myself.

When food was out of the question, I only had purses, shoes, and makeup left as rewards. This worked for a while. Most girls know this all too well; I think it might even be a chapter in the girl handbook. I can't even tell you how many authors I know who buy a new handbag whenever they release a book. It's so popular that I've even overheard a group of authors discussing it at a conference.

This can become a bit of an issue when you've released nearly one hundred books in five years—that's a lot of closet space, and when you're a family of eight, closet space is hard to come by. I do enjoy a nice large bag, as my YOU CAN DO IT FACEBOOK GROUP can tell you, because I'm often telling them how great bags are for carrying your snacks on the go. But, in reality, there are only so many material things you can have before it becomes too much.

I was on a quest to figure out the best ways to love myself. When I did some evaluation, I realized that having some me-time was often what really refreshed me and helped me recenter and regroup.

Me-time is a bit hard to come by in our household. And I

also knew that when I had time to myself, I used it to work. It was very, very difficult for me to put work or other responsibilities aside and take care of myself.

I made the physical aspect of taking care of myself a priority, and taking time to run or workout became part of my self-care routine. But I needed a mental component as well. Journaling, meditation, and prayer were the first ways I did this. I can't tell you what a difference this made for me in every single area of my life. It's been amazing!

When I took my Enneagram evaluation and found out I was a four, it made even more sense for me to make self-care a priority. Fours need solitude and silence, but I NEVER HAD IT! This is also why I think I often felt as if the world was moving so fast, that everything was so loud and too much. Making space for alone time in the mornings really brought my mental needs to the forefront.

How many of us mamas enjoy any time alone, as in *really* alone and *truly* quiet? I know I almost never did. Even if I did get a second to myself, I didn't spend it on self-evaluation or meditation.

This might sound like a luxury to many of you; I get it. I know some of you might be thinking that even if you did wake up early, or set aside some time for yourself in the evening, there are about twenty other things you should be doing instead. Those ten to twenty minutes of me-time seem like time you just don't have to give. I know what you are facing. But what this past year has taught me is that I *have* to carve out time for things like self-care. The difference in how I deal with stress, how I interact with my kids, how I sleep, and how I live has changed drastically from this simple act.

Another thing that's been huge for me is finding something I love or have always wanted to do and DOING IT. Jack and I realized I needed a hobby. I know our situation is unique, and not everyone works from home like I do, but during the winter last year I realized I had to be able to leave the house, even if it was just once a week or, heck, once every other week. I didn't even know what I wanted to do when I left the house, but I knew it had to be something for my mind and body, and it had to be something just for me.

This was hard, because carving out time for myself seemed selfish. Our family schedule is always so packed; if one of my kids wanted to try soccer or an art class I'd make it work, but when it came to setting aside time for me, it was much harder to do. Like 99 percent of other moms, I usually put everything and everyone before myself. When I started achieving my health goals and realizing I had some mental and emotional work to do, the ways I *didn't* love myself floated up to the surface. I wasn't very kind to myself. Why? I actually talked to my counselor about this: I'm *so* hard on myself. I realized that when I thought about doing things for myself, I actually felt weak. I thought that not only *couldn't* I do it, but I *shouldn't* do it.

I thought about the many things I wanted to do—I would love to tap again; I've always wanted to paint; I wanted to try paddle boarding. I even considered taking a fancy bread-making class. I offered up these ideas to my counselor and she suggested I add a meditation or yoga class to the list. That sounded a bit boring, but I added it anyway. Guess what I ended up doing? I know, I know, right? The most boring of all... meditation and yoga. I really wasn't 100 percent sold on it, but I trusted her, and felt like maybe this would be really good for me.

I found a yoga class close to our home that I attend every other week for an hour, and I do this all by myself. It has been an amazing experience, even life-changing. The yoga part of the class is mostly stretching, which is amazing for muscles that are so often a tight, knotted-up mess. I get to focus on my breathing, and I clear my mind. I can't imagine my life without it now.

The first few times I went to class were very challenging, and I had a mental block about it. Part of this was because I'm a workaholic—it was super hard not to think about how I should be working instead. I also had a hard time leaving the house to do something that seemed like such a luxury. Added to this were questions like who will be there? Will it be weird? I'm so awkward. Will I do a pose and either fall over or fart? It's crazy the sort of crazy ideas we conjure up when trying something new. But once I got past those first weeks, the class became something I looked forward to.

Why is it so hard for us as women—and especially as mothers—to do this sort of thing when we so desperately need it? This class only cost what two Starbucks would, so I could have found a way to do this for myself even when my kids were little, but I think there are simply times in our lives when we ignore the things we need because we're just surviving.

I had decided I needed not only to survive, but thrive, and this required different choices and purposeful self-care.

> There is always a choice. You can do it. You just have to figure out a way to make it important, to make *you* important.

This is how it looked for me, and I'm grateful that my work with fasting caused me to really look at this part of my life so I could make these changes. I honestly think if I hadn't tried fasting I would still be rewarding myself in the same old ways, and the different aspects of how I wasn't taking care of myself wouldn't have come into view.

I am not sure where you are in your journey. I'm not sure if this even applies to you. Maybe you've always been one of those women who did self-care naturally, but I'm guessing there are a few women out there who need to hear this. It's important to do this stuff. It doesn't have to take time away from your family, work, marriage, or other important responsibilities and relationships, and honestly, those things will even benefit from it. I have no idea how this will look in your life; it might look a lot like what I needed, or it might just be one small little tweak to what you're already doing. Maybe you just need to get up a few minutes earlier and open up a devotional. Maybe you need to join a local cooking class or take time to hike or bike each week. There are no set rules here, you just have to look outside a reward system that revolves around material things, or rewards that you eat and drink.

> You deserve a reward that lasts, a reward that continues to help you and heal you.

During the first meditation class I ever attended the teacher said that our minds are like little birds searching for a branch to land upon. I started to cry when I heard this. YES! That described my mind exactly. My mind was a bird looking for a place to rest and, let me tell you, ladies, doing this meditation and stretching is a branch for me. It has been such a gift to me that I honestly wish I could just grab all of you and drag you with me to my class.

My mind had been fluttering along for so long. Once I realized that, and really embraced the idea that I needed to get quiet and delve inside myself a bit and really get things in order, it was a bit of a revelation. I realized that many of us reach far outside ourselves and become loud in an attempt to fill that huge, hurting, empty hole inside of us.

One of the other things that these meditations really helped me with was connecting my mind to my belly! This was HUGE! My amazing teacher said our bellies are the place where we digest everything, even mental, emotional, and spiritual things. Doesn't it make sense, then, that so many of us fill that hole of pain with food to try and digest what has happened to us in our lives? Once we're conscious of our choices and our body, things fall in line and we can become whole again.

Mindfulness meditation has been such a beautiful blessing in my life that just thinking about it makes me want to cry. I think about my little five-year-old self who was so confused about food, and so innocent. When I'm meditating, I hug her. She's a fighter and I'm so proud of her.

I would love you to think about a point in your life that needs a hug, and do it. Close your eyes and visualize the pain or the trauma, or the times when you couldn't take care of yourself the way you really should have. Hug that precious girl. Hug her tight. Hold her.

You were loved then and you are loved now.

You were perfect then and you are perfect now. Just keep holding on to her and walk forward.

She's with you on this journey and she's proud of you, too.

MY FAVORITE KINDS OF SELF-CARE

- A nice long, hot bath with my waterproof kindle, bubbles, and a glass of dry red wine.
- A walk along the beach with Jack.
- Yoga. For yoga at home, try the Yoga Studio app—it's amazing!
- Journaling, prayer, and meditation.
- Coffee in the morning while watching the sunrise.
- Going out by myself to a movie, the library, or the park.
- Going for a walk or run.
- Riding my horse or snuggling with the animals.
- Taking a class or going to a retreat

What can you do for yourself today that's loving and kind?

The Importance of Support

T his past year, as I've been involved in my one-on-one coaching, I've seen over and over again how important it is to have support is on your wellness journey. The women who tend to have an easier time with counseling are the ones who have a solid support system set up. They have a husband, a mother, a sister, a friend, or a coworker they can turn to. Some of the ladies have an Internet buddy who they teamed up with in my Facebook group. It doesn't really matter who the person is, or how they got together, although I will say that having someone in your home is most ideal.

The ladies who don't have someone to share their journey with often seem to struggle a little more with things. I hear how alone they feel, or there is someone in their home who makes fun of them or even sabotages their progress. It was so sad for me to see these women and know how hard it was for them to overcome the negativity they were experiencing every day. One of them in particular was nearly in tears with me talking about how her family made fun of almost anything she ate. This is horrible! I've suggested to all of these women that they make a plea online in my FB group to find someone to befriend who will support them on their journey. Even one person we can talk to about our health changes will make a huge difference.

I know it's easy for me to tell you not to listen to the naysayers in your home, especially when you know how supportive my family has been to me. I know many of you have people in your family who say nasty things to you, which not only causes you stress, but it makes you think you won't be able to do this. Please, don't believe them! My best advice is to try and journal about it, speak positively to yourself, and try as best you can to not to let them get to you.

The best medicine I've found for proving these people wrong is through your success. When your family members start to see changes happening in you, it'll be much more difficult for them to bring you down about what you're doing wrong. Remember—the only person you can control in this situation is you! Continue to be positive and eventually you might win that person over and show them that making better choices for themselves will be good too. I've seen this happen in a few of the families in my group. There was one woman in particular who endured negativity for over a year before the other people in the family were finally convinced about her process to achieve wellness. They finally jumped on board by supporting her, and even started making their own changes. There is hope! Don't despair.

With fasting, my advice is usually to keep the fact that you're fasting to yourself unless you want to hear lots of reasons why you shouldn't do it. Frankly, there's a stigma attached to fasting, and right now people tend to think it's a fad, that it's trendy. If you're looking for support it might be best to reach out to someone who has mentioned they were interested in fasting, or who has tried a fast. Maybe you have a friend who has told you she would like to try fasting, or maybe one of your friends has been working on a similar plan and might be interested in talking with you about your health changes. I don't think they need to even necessarily be on the exact same plan as you, but having someone who will understand your need for encouragement will make a big difference to your progress.

I remember being a kid attending Weight Watchers meetings. My favorite part of the meeting was when someone would share that they had reached a certain goal and everyone would clap and cheer for that person. I thought it was so cool to join in the celebration when someone achieved their goal. Unfortunately, I'm not able to do this in person with the ladies and gentlemen in my group, but we love to do it virtually. If you've been following my plan, I highly suggest joining our group and sharing your success with us. I know I say it in every book, but that group is seriously the most positive and supportive collection of humans on the planet. Everyone is a cheerleader. Ladies across the globe have celebrated each other's successes and achievements—races completed, sizes down, pregnancy, medication no longer needed. We've seen so many awesome things happen. I've also seen that those who share often are also the ones who see consistent, positive changes with their health. I know it can be scary to put yourself out there, but there are rewards to opening up and letting people support and encourage you. Don't be afraid, just ask.

> You can find the group HERE.:
> m.facebook.com/groups/957213331029100

I've also been happy to see several women in my group simply asking those around them at work or church if they wanted to join up to get healthier together using my plan. How awesome is that? We even have one group in Ohio and another in Colorado that are twenty-plus members strong. These groups have lost hundreds of pounds together while meeting weekly or biweekly for support and encouragement and to trade recipes. I love it!

Maybe you could put up a flier in your library, or church, or at work. Or maybe you have a friend who has mentioned they want to find someone to walk with, or you could start up a healthy meal club where you all get together and make healthy #wilderway freezer meals to share. The possibilities are endless.

One of the things that I have been working on a lot this past year is hospitality. God laid it on my heart to invite people over for dinner. So far we've invited three families to join us for dinner, and although it can be a lot of work, we've enjoyed using our home and our meals to show people they are loved.

Maybe you have a meal or special healthy treat that everyone raves about—make that meal or treat, open your door, invite people in, and start a conversation with them about food—you might even find local friends who want to try the same thing. The food and health revolution is through mother to child, wife to husband, and friend to friend.

Another awesome idea that one of my #wilderway ladies emailed me about was a walking/wogging club they had started at their local elementary school. They just walk, wog, or jog one or two days a week after they drop the kids off at school. That sounds so fun! I wish they all lived closer to me so I could join them. Just imagine how cool it will be years from now when these ladies can look back on their journey together, how many steps they've walked together while talking about their kids, their health, and their goals!

Finding a group of friends, or even one good friend, to join you on this journey, or just having someone who can encourage you along the way can make the difference between success and failure. I hope you're able to find someone who makes it easier for you to reach your goals. I think it's so beautiful to see families making these changes together. My hope and prayer is that these changes will continue for generations to come.

We can do it together!

PART 3

The Life Of A Faster

(AKA JASINDA'S FASTING JOURNALS)

OVER THE NEXT HALF OF THE BOOK I'M GOING TO SHARE my personal experiences about fasting with you. Some of these adventures are extremely personal and probably shouldn't even be shared, but I figure if I can share something—even something personal—that can help someone, I should. I'm going to be honest with you. If you get to a part that's TMI for you it's okay…just pass over it and keep going. I'm going to start at the beginning of last year and just keep on rocking out my experiences for you so that if you get stuck, or discouraged, or frustrated you can look back and see that I made it through and YOU CAN TOO!

April 2017—Prior to this time I had only dabbled in fasting. I would clean fast until lunch or even wait to eat until later in the afternoon, usually around 2-3 p.m. Jack and I were experimenting with working out while fasting—more on this later—so we would work out in a fasted state in the morning and then delay eating for a few hours. It honestly wasn't difficult for us as long as we had coffee.

Warm liquids seemed to be key for me with fasting. If we didn't have something hot like coffee, tea, or even just hot water in the morning, fasting was much more difficult for both of us. Another key ingredient for me was Pure LaCroix. If I didn't have some carbonated, flavorless water for fasting, it was also much more difficult. I think having something going through the body, especially carbonation, can help you feel less empty and give your body a bit more "movement."

> I'm also going to repeat that salt was and still is a key component to my fasting. If I start feeling weird, icky, shaky, hangry, or just not my usual ball of sunshine self, I suck on some salt.

I know some people freak out about salt, but I've read entire books on salt and I can tell you that if you should be concerned about salt it's the stuff you see on most dining room tables. If we're talking about pink Himalayan salt, mineral salts, or other sea salts, you have nothing to worry about. I've even seen a lack of salt cause some health issues. Frequent Headaches? Try some salt. When you're drinking as much water as most people do when they fast, that salt is going to flush right through you. If you have questions on this then consult your doctor, but don't be surprised if they say I'm crazy. I doubt many doctors are reading about salt, but you might have a really good one who does. Usually when I talk to my doctors, they're learning more from me on these sorts of nutritional topics than I am from them. What I've learned from my doctors is that they just don't have the time or the opportunity to study nutrition because they're busy keeping up with medicine. I think it's just the nature of the beast with the medical profession right now.

I really hope to see this change.

We have to stop chasing the symptoms in medical practice and start treating the actual problem with a real, viable cure; that's just my two cents as someone whose symptoms have been treated with medicine unsuccessfully for my entire life.

Back to April 2017: I decided I wanted to try a longer extended fast. As I said earlier, I liked the idea of this being a spiritual endeavor as well as a healthful one, and I really wanted to work on autophagy for some skin issues I was having—again more on that later—so I knew I needed to fast for at least three days totally clean. I also wanted to use this time to monitor my blood sugars during the fast. Would they shoot up like I had heard they might, or would they go down? Would they go too low?

I had lots of questions so I figured now was as good a time as any to try and figure it out. What was the worst that would happen? If I didn't feel good, I would eat.

An important side note here is that one of my biggest concerns was not being able to eat with my family. I actually contacted a doctor who specializes in therapeutic fasting and we had several conversations about this. I knew my kids would have questions about this and I wanted to be able to answer their questions openly and honestly. Also, I wasn't sure if, starting out, I would be strong enough to prepare or serve dinner to them on an empty stomach. Was I going to be able to sit with them at the table as they were eating? To make things even more complicated, my family does a devotional and special share time about our day during dinner. I *really* felt it was important to be there for that. I decided I would just try it out and see if there was a good way for me to participate and be around to enjoy our usual family routines. Heck, I was even worried about making lunches for my kids. Would I be okay around food at all? I was assured that this is more challenging when you're starting with longer fasts, but that it *does* get better as you go and will eventually not be an issue at all.

I was still unsure. Again, this is all a head game. These are real and authentic thoughts, but they're often what stops us from even trying, and from being successful.

Get out of your head and in the game! You don't know if you can do it until you try.

DAY 1: (OF AN ATTEMPTED 3–5 DAY WATER FAST)

I started the fast at 10 p.m. the previous evening, after a 5 p.m.-10 p.m. eating window.

The first thing I did after I woke up the following morning was to grab some warm liquid.

> IMPORTANT REMINDER: you need to keep tea and coffee plain and unsweetened so you don't raise insulin and break your fast! You don't want to break your fast! Don't do it! I usually have one or two cups of coffee, and follow it up with a cup or two of tea. Yes, this means I pee all morning long, but warm fluids make me so happy.

The morning is actually surprisingly easy. I sucked on a little bit of salt at the end of the morning, but I was surprised by how little I needed. I'm feeling pretty good. Afternoon is a bit more difficult. I have another cup of tea and then head right for some LaCroix. Yes, I am literally in the bathroom ALL DAY LONG. I'm just learning to be okay with it. Still feeling pretty good. Dinnertime is rough. I can't sit with the family during dinner, and I think about breaking my fast. Ugh, it will get better, right? We do our sharing and devotional time away from the table tonight and the kids don't enjoy it as much as when we sit at the table, but we made it work. Karri says she will make the kids' lunches for me.

I have to be honest and say this evening is pretty rough. I have lots of thoughts about breaking my fast. Even SPAM with a side of mushrooms is sounding good to me. Heck, even the dog food smells a bit appetizing. I'm losing it. Time for bed!

DAY 2:

Woke up feeling really good! I was going to try warm water this morning, but I'm worried about a headache with the crazy day I have lined up, so I think I need coffee. I'll try just water tomorrow.

The day goes pretty easy. Again, better than I expected… #winning

I did have a silly amount of coffee and tea, but I made it

through and that's what counts. Afternoon was better than yesterday and again I did SOS—suck on salt—whenever I wasn't feeling my usual stellar self. I think I ended up needing more salt today, but not an insane amount.

Okay, so I lied: might be a little crazy how much salt I'm taking. When we get to dinnertime, I really need my salt. I tried to sit with the family when they were eating. I'm not going to lie—it was HARD, but I did it. I had a LaCroix while they ate. I've told the kids I'm fasting to try and heal my body. They seemed okay with it after I explained, but my littlest boy really still wanted me to eat, so I sat with them and sipped and sipped, but it still made me a little sad.

Again, I think about breaking my fast. It seems like it would be so much easier. Maybe this is a dumb idea...I'm totally second-guessing myself, but I'm almost forty-eight hours in and autophagy has hopefully kicked in and I really want to do this. I CAN DO THIS!

Jack cleared the table and made lunches (he's a saint), and I keep going. Tomorrow I will feel better! Tomorrow, tomorrow! I can make it to tomorrow!

I go to bed with more salt and my LaCroix. Okay, actually I had two LaCroix. I know I'm going to be up ALL NIGHT going to the bathroom. YIKES! Yep, peeing all night. I have the bladder of a miniature squirrel.

Note to self: don't drink all the LaCroix before bed.

Additional note to self: Why did I think this was a good idea?

DAY 3:

So in the fasting world everyone says Day 3 is a magical point, and I have to say I agree. I'm drinking water only this morning! I'm a bit worried about getting a caffeine headache, but I think it will be worth it to try. I've read that to get the full benefit of autophagy I need to drink water only, so I owe it to myself to at least try. Midmorning I almost cave and have some coffee or tea. I'm definitely getting a caffeine headache.

SOS! SOS! SOS! I grab some salt and pray for the best.

Worst-case scenario I'll have some tea.

Headache is worse in the afternoon.

Note to self: wean myself off caffeine *first* next time. This is just dumb—DUMB.

SOS!

I almost break down and have coffee when Jack has some in the afternoon, but I'm strong and I resist. I take a bath instead; I've heard that taking a bath with some salts is also really good during a fast, and I have to agree. I feel really good getting out of the bath. I just have to make it through dinner and I'm halfway through this.

Dinner is actually doable today and although the kids are asking again why I can't eat and I need to explain it again, everyone seems to be getting more used to the idea. They aren't totally okay with me not eating, but they understand. Jack still thinks I might be actually crazy, but I feel and look good today. I even had a stranger tell me that my skin was glowing—weird! My cheeks do seem a bit pink, though, and the other strange thing I'm experiencing is that it feels like my skin is tightening. Hard to explain, but it really feels like my body is lighter too.

TMI warning: I've only pooped twice since starting this, but I think I'm totally empty or close to empty so that might have something to do with feeling "light." I'm excited to see how I feel tomorrow.

Only one LaCroix before bed tonight and I slept like a baby.

DAY 4:

I can honestly say I'm no longer hungry. I'm down a handful of pounds and I feel like a million bucks! I even did a short workout with weights this morning. Yes, that's how good I feel.

I wrote ALL THE WORDS TODAY! I'm still just doing water and my headache is totally gone. I've been taking lots of salt but not insane amounts—just a normal amount for a woman who hasn't had any real food in four days. I know, I know, I sound crazy.

Dinner is the only time I actually struggle today. The kids really want me to eat. Ugh, the little ones just don't understand. We keep talking about it. We've discussed how it's helping me heal; this is a constant discussion with my kids. We talk about my health and always have; the content of the conversation just keeps changing. My older kids get it but the little ones are still questioning. I hope at some point my little kids will understand better. I know that the older kids see that I don't need to nap anymore, that food isn't making me sick, and that I'm more active with them. I knew it would just take time and I think these conversations are good.

I try not to hide my struggles from them in the hopes that it will make them stronger as they grow and face difficult things. I talk to them about how good I'm feeling right now, and it helps. I help with packing lunches tonight and really don't even have the urge to eat.

I have one LaCroix before bed as Jack and I watch a show and I wake up raring to go!

DAY 5:

I literally wake up feeling like I could run a marathon. I feel like I'm actually floating and it feels amazing. I can't believe I haven't had any food in five days! This is pure craziness!

I try to visualize all of the food I might have eaten this week.

I honestly feel like I could go on with this for another five days. I'm not going to, but I feel like I *could*. I plan to break my fast this evening and then enjoy the holiday weekend celebrating with my family. I really doubted some of the things I've read about fasting, such as some people start to feel nearly superhuman once they reach a certain point, but I'm actually feeling that way. Yes, I have moments where I feel a bit "off" but as soon as I SOS, it goes away. I'm still drinking ALL THE

LACROIX, but at this point I can go much longer without it. I've found that if I drink it out of a straw I seem to drink it more slowly than when if I drink it out of a can. I bought a cool cup at Starbucks that's really big and has sparkles and fits two full cans, and I look awesome sipping out of it. No, really, I do.

Around five I decide to break my fast with a few handfuls of nuts, and I'm immediately in the bathroom. I guess I wasn't empty. Next time, I'm going to try something else—I hear pickles and olives are good. After another hour, and two trips to the bathroom, I decide to try some salad and that sits better. THANK THE LORD!

My family eats together about 7 p.m., and I don't eat much this evening but I'm still feeling good. My kids are *so* happy mama is eating. My youngest son who had the biggest issues with me not eating is literally holding on to me while we eat. He's just the sweetest little thing and he's ecstatic to be near me while we eat. This has really shown me how freaking important the social aspect of eating together as a family is.

I know I've talked about it in other books, but we really try to make dinnertime special in our family. We light candles and dim the lights, and we'll play classical or jazz music if we want to make things really special—usually when we eat at home on the weekends. #sofancy I learned this trick early on as the best way to set a calm, peaceful tone at dinner so my crazy kids won't be so darn crazy during dinner. IT WORKS.

After dinner I decide to have a glass of red wine to celebrate and that one glass hits me *hard*. Please, be careful with this. I honestly feel like I've had two or three glasses when I've only had one. This reduced consumption might help with our wine budget, but I could see it as potentially dangerous too.

Note to self: DON'T BREAK AN EXTENDED FAST WITH WINE!

Overall I felt this fast was very successful, so much so that I saw a physical change in my body almost immediately. I do think I ate a bit more than normal for the two days after my fast, but I actually think it's really important for revving the metabolism back up. I did spend a full five days fasting, so it only makes sense to do a few days of feasting as well. During those two days of eating after my fast, I regained about half of the weight I lost through the fast. BUT it's important to note that my body composition stayed the same, meaning that I was losing OLD fat. The weight that I put back on was most likely water, and not fat.

I think this is really, *really* important to remember. Some of this "old fat" is going to be a bear to get off and that's why I think fasting works so well toward the end of your weight-loss journey. Our ten or twenty or even thirty-year-old fat, like mine, will not want to leave easily. I can promise you that. Old fat is happy fat. It's been sitting all nice and dense for ages and it isn't going to want to leave until you give it a going-away party with a printed invitation. That is what fasting is for that final ten to twenty pounds: it's a ticket to ride, an invitation to the final dance, the last big hurrah.

Right after this fast Jack and I had an event and I decided to fast during that travel time. We fasted for the twenty-four hours it took us to get to the event city and we fasted through the event itself. We had an amazing meal afterward. That was the first time I had ever fasted during an event, so I was a bit nervous about my stamina. Usually an event takes a lot out of me, but I was actually really focused and full of energy. For those of you who might be worried about working while fasting, I really do think it can be done. I wouldn't suggest having a really stressful work event or meeting at the height of hunger (usually between eighteen to twenty hours into a fast), but I think it's totally fine to experiment and see where your comfort levels are.

I also want to quickly touch on the mental and spiritual benefits I felt from this 5-day fast. If you take a look at all of the major spiritual teachers—Jesus, Muhammad, and Buddha—they all agreed on one thing: fasting. I don't think you even need to be a very spiritual person to receive something spiritual from the practice of fasting.

When you fast you'll find your head is "clearer" and, your productivity will increase without even trying. This works especially well for me because it creates time for my spiritual life, which is so easy for me to forget about when my mind isn't as focused. I've made the space for prayer, journaling, and meditation when I've given up food, and God gives me a spiritual space with him I often neglect otherwise.

I struggle with a bit of ADHD, and when my mind is

being pulled in a million different directions I feel like my connection to God is subsequently lessened. When I'm fasting I don't feel that same way; I think this is because there's such a strong body and mind connection—when our body is able to function more effectively, it opens the mind in a way that I believe is by intentional design.

Our bodies weren't made to digest 24-7, hence the term "breaking fast", and I think if you look at how humans hunted and gathered, with natural seasons of harvest and seasons of scarcity, it makes sense that our minds sharpen when food isn't as readily available so we can continue to survive. God designed us this way—we are designed to survive periods of time without food.

Our modern culture of convenience means food is available everywhere all the time. We can't walk two steps without seeing a vending machine, a giant poster of the newest fast-food craze, or a 1,000 calorie coffee concoction. It's just the era we live in. This is a blessing and a curse, but for such a sedentary society, this creates quite an issue. We're eating all the time and sitting on our butts in front of screens all day long. Honestly I think it might be a miracle that we aren't all 500 lbs!

When we live, eat, play, work, love, and rest in the way God designed, we find the greatest rewards in life. I've found so much healing in this. When we work *with* our body instead of *against* it, we receive both mental healing as well as physical healing. So much of my prayer journal reflects this. Instead of just doing things the way society dictates, I think and reflect on the way God would want me to live, and try to understand his plan for me. I know that this doesn't necessarily gel with everyone who is reading this, but it's important for me to touch on it because it's such a large part of my journey and story.

I know it might shock some people to read about my spiritual practices because of the fictional content of my books, but I *assure* you God knows all about that too. Don't worry: GOD KNOWS JASINDA LIKES SEX. LOL!

> My best advice for you if you're looking for a spiritual component to your fasting is to pray, journal, and meditate. And when I say meditate I mostly mean sit, be quiet, and listen. You might still hear your own thoughts, but if you can just sit in silence and stillness for at least three minutes, you'll probably hear something from outside of yourself, and that's the good stuff. Create those moments for yourself on a daily basis and you'll reap *so* much from fasting.

Fasting has been better for me than any drug, wine, or tropical vacation. If my mind isn't in a good place, I've found it can be nearly impossible to be my best self and be fully present. There are so many gifts to be found in rest, solitude, and quiet.

I didn't do an extended fast again for a month, but I did continue to experiment with window fasting, intermittent fasting, and every other day fasting.

JUNE 2017

DAY 1 OF AN ATTEMPTED 7–DAY EXTENDED FAST:

So in June we were traveling again and I decided I wanted to do another extended fast, specifically to work on autophagy.

As you may remember from my other books, I've had continued issues with hanging skin in the lower half of my body. In the summer months, this gets much worse, sometimes even leading to infection. I've met with a plastic surgeon several times to discuss it, but I always chicken out because of my increasing number of scars, as well as the high risk of infection, and this particular surgery involves a very difficult recovery. We've discussed a modification of the most common surgical procedure, and a month ago I met with another surgeon to discuss it. I probably just need more time, but at this point it still isn't something I'm ready to do until I've exhausted all other options…so autophagy it is!

The hardest part for me with these long fasts isn't actually not eating, but rather the lack of caffeine, so with this fast I'm going to try and wean myself off the caffeine or lower my dependency on the caffeine by using some caffeinated water versus the hot liquids I'm so very addicted to.

We usually do brunch on Sunday, so I decided I would load up on bacon and eggs at brunch and then fast from there. Brunch with my family is one of our favorite pastimes: we go to church on Sunday morning and then right after church we go to a local restaurant for brunch and eat *all the things*. We're so lucky that they always have bacon, eggs, and berries, because those are in our family's list of top-ten foods. My little baby daughter loves berries so much she has, on occasion, overindulged nearly to the point of illness. I swear she could eat her actual weight in blueberries! They also have some wonderful cream I pour into my coffee that's a great fat to indulge in before fasting. I had some cream, bacon, sausage, eggs in oil, berries, more bacon, and champagne. It was wonderful and amazing!

At the time I thought this was the perfect plan, but I quickly discovered that following brunch by starting my fast was hellish. I had to watch everyone else eat dinner that evening, and I couldn't go to sleep as I usually would. To top it off, packing lunches was pure torture. I think, for me at least, it's easier to start a fast *after* dinner and then go to bed, as opposed to having brunch and then fasting for the remainder of the day. I hated it, but I stuck with it. I almost caved, but I did manage to hold it together.

It sucks to go to bed craving food, so I sucked down two LaCroixs right before bed...which made me need to pee all night. Why didn't I remember that this never goes well?

Note to self: NO GUZZLING WATER BEFORE BED.

DAY 2:

We're traveling most of the day today, so it should be fairly easy, right? Wrong. I drank my weight in coffee. Total fail. I thought I could handle having only water since I'd been weaning myself, but the travel just required the lovely, life-giving liquid known as coffee. I just *had* to have it. I am so weak. Gah! I did also SOS a lot, probably every hour. So... loads of salt and tons of coffee. I did have lots of water when the family stopped for dinner, but then I had to stop and pee every hour for three hours after that, which was pure torture, although traveling with six kids might also be torture on its own.

> Important note: I'm really not into torturing myself...okay maybe I am a tiny bit, but it was exaggerated by traveling with our whole crew PLUS hitting the height of hunger at the point of greatest stress. I don't recommend this. Please learn from my mistakes.

The great thing is, when I think about these extended fasts, intermittent fasting and window fasting are an absolute joy.

DAY 3:

Today was much easier. I was able to stick to mostly water and salt. We will arrive at our first destination today and everyone is in a much better mood. I'm excited to see how I feel tomorrow. I'm going for water only!

DAYS 4 AND DAY 5:

These days were very similar so I'm combining them. I was able to stick to water and I swear I could feel some skin tightening, mostly in my stomach area, not my lower half. I haven't needed as much sleep as usual. I am running on about six hours versus my usual eight. I'm in no mood to work out, but I'm feeling really well.

DAY 6:

Today was the event, and I decided to eat afterward. I didn't get as far with my fast as I wanted, but I just knew my body needed food. It's important to note it wasn't that I couldn't go on because I wasn't feeling well, but rather that I missed the social aspect and joy of eating. You all know I preach no deprivation, and usually during my fasts I really don't feel that way, but today I did and so I decided to eat. As I've said before, this should be fluid and flexible: when you feel the need to eat you should probably eat. Six days was enough for this one and now I'm going to enjoy the remainder of my vacation with my family.

It's also super important to note that usually in the few days after I break my fast I ate mostly all gray plates. This is actually contrary to the prevailing wisdom on fasting because most of the doctors who do therapeutic fasting also say to stick to a ketogenic (think Black plate) type meal because it makes it much easier to go into another period of fasting.

When you have healthy carbs, the water weight increases more quickly, but after an extended fast I want to FEAST, so I allow myself some low glycemic carbs. In fact, I've haven't seen it make much difference to my blood sugar; I monitored my blood sugar during my fasts, and it remained steady. My body feels great, and I think my metabolism has ignited a bit. Some health and nutrition people would call this a "carb up," but I just call it my happiest eating days. These are the days when you'll catch me eating a peanut butter and jelly on toasted sprouted bread, or some Greek yogurt with pecans and dark chocolate.

I get excited just thinking about it! Although, to be fair, it doesn't take much to get me excited these days.

JULY AND AUGUST

These two months were mostly window fasting with a few 24- or 36-hour fasts thrown in. I didn't do ANY fasting on the weekends at all, and I continued to indulge in wonderful things like beer, wine, Halo Top ice cream, glorious #wilderway s'mores, and avocados on sprouted toast. I've decided summer isn't a season of fasting for me; summer is about family and food and beaches and beer and popcorn. The fun part is that I really haven't gained any weight during this time. My usual ten-pound weight fluctuation still happens, but my body composition has pretty much stayed the same.

I've continued to do my quick workouts with weights, or

my own bodyweight, for maybe twenty minutes three times a week, but I haven't been running much at all. We've been swimming and playing together as a family, so my workouts have been much less because I'm just trying to enjoy the warm months with my family—and I LOVE IT! I've also probably had too many gluten-free pizzas while sitting out on the deck of our favorite local pizza joints, but guess what? I'm okay with that too. I'm enjoying it and I'm enjoying this time together with my family while enjoying my favorite foods. No guilt here, only grace.

Around this same time we found a large lump in my leg. We had several consults, hospital visits, and x-rays, and it was determined that this lump was "fossilized" fat. You guys! My fat is so old it's turning into a fossil! I'm not even kidding. My doctor said they usually only find these sorts of masses in breast tissue, and that it should stay put unless and until it becomes painful. I agreed with her and will keep my fossil fat for now, keeping an eye on it and reporting any changes.

SEPTEMBER

DAYS 1–5 OF A 5-DAY FAST:

After the fossil fat incident, I decided I wanted to keep trying for autophagy. Jack and I had another event coming up and I decided to attempt a clean water fast so I could make some progress on my legs. I decided I just had to get down to business with this attempt at autophagy; it was my will versus my skin and the fossil fat rock. I was determined AF! Watch out!

I hate to call this fast easy… but it was seriously *easy*. I'm not sure if it was because the kids were all back in school, or that I was just in the right frame of mind, or that I was just ready to do it because my fasting muscle was more developed. Whatever the reason, it was pretty darn easy.

Jack and I arrived at our event and I decided to break my fast with a delicious seafood dinner. It was SO GOOD! And then I felt so good that whole week! I had that glow and float feeling for most of the week, and about 90 percent of my liquid intake was water only. I didn't see much progress with leg skin, but I did feel a tightening in my core. Again, I'm not really sure why my torso is in the skin tightening game and my lower body is not—maybe it's just gravity, but my legs just don't seem to be making any progress. I'm not giving up on it yet, if only because I've seen other people take a solid year with extended fasting before they see improvement. As far as autophagy goes, I'm seeing some definite improvement in my face, so I know it's working; it's nothing shocking, but I think I'll see more improvement over time.

I admit it's hard to hold on to hope with this process when I don't see anything much happening but, regardless, I'm going to cling to the small amount of hope I have that I will see some improvement eventually. I know it's healing my body in other ways. The skin on my neck is showing some improvement, for one thing, and I get daily comments about my skin "glowing."

The other amazing thing is that since I've been fasting my nutritional counts have continued to go up! So much so that my hematologist is going to let me remove my port! THIS IS AMAZING NEWS, GUYS! I've had my port for NINE YEARS! It's been the champion of all ports for me, but it was getting past the point where it should still be inside of me. Either I had to get my counts stabilized, or we would have to put in a new port.

At this point in my surgical life, the thought of having to have another port was so depressing. I was so fearful my counts would drop again, and I honestly think my doctor was too. He had been clear when he said he wanted to see a full year of good reports before he would even discuss taking it out. When he finally agreed I could get it out I was so excited I was literally jumping with joy. It's hard to explain unless you've had a port, but I had been living with the irritation of it for so long that I was overwhelmed with the thought of not having it any longer. I couldn't or wouldn't wear clothes that exposed it, to the point that I even had flowers sewn onto my matron of honor dress for my sister's wedding because it bothered me so much.

I'm sure not everyone who has a port is as bothered by it as I was, but mine was very large and often tipped especially when I was sleeping, so the idea of not having to deal with that was RADICAL! PRAISE THE LORD! This was an indicator to me that the fasting was not only working on the outside, but also on the inside. I wasn't losing a ton of weight, but I just LOOKED so freaking healthy! I was really starting to see more muscle definition in my arms even though I was working out less, and I felt *so* good. Like, better than I ever have in my life.

The other amazing thing is that I didn't have any sudden drops or rises in my blood sugar. I would occasionally get spikes or dips before, but now it was steadily in a normal range, which was another indication that good things were happening. I think my insulin resistance was almost totally healed. Again, PTL.

If you've had issues with insulin resistance, blood sugar, inflammation, skin sag or other skin issues, gut problems, gluten intolerance…and nearly anything else, I really think trying some internment fasting might help. Recent studies are showing that a 3-day fast can totally reset your immunity.

Google it if you don't believe me.

OCTOBER AND NOVEMBER

I tried to do a 24- or 36-hour fast every week during the autumn. Some weeks I didn't fast at all, and some weeks I did three days in a row. Some days I fasted every other day, and some weeks I did black plate days and then fasted for two days, followed by another day of black plates. It honestly just depended on how I was feeling. I didn't go any longer than three days, because that really seems to be a sweet spot for me. I was also getting to a good place with my weight and was getting into a groove with our daily routine. I believe if things aren't broke, don't fix it. I also continued to live it up on the weekend, enjoying my gray plate weekend lifestyle. Man, I just love that.

I also stopped working out on the weekend unless we were doing a fun family run. I'm sticking to a quick and dirty workout of maybe twenty minutes three days a week and, honestly, this is all I want to do or have time to do. Another cool—well, hot, actually—thing that Jack and I have been doing is exercising under infrared lights in a sauna. This really helps with our sleep issues, considering our constant exposure to white screens. You can find cheap red light bulbs on Amazon, so you can try this even if you don't have a sauna. It will be a shock to your body, but it *so* good for you. Think of hot yoga but hotter—*wink-wink*.

So, these things all added up to great rest, great feasting, great fasting, great playtime, and great work time. I also carved out time each morning so I could journal and pray. This does take some effort to manage, but it's worth it to me, and I believe everything in my life is better because of it.

JASINDA'S SUPER QUICK AND DIRTY DAILY BODY WEIGHT WORKOUT:

- 20 squats or 10 jump squats depending on how I'm feeling that day
- 20 leg raises
- 20 bench dips

- 20 jumping jacks
- 20 pushups
- 1-minute plank

Repeat until you're spent. I usually rest a few minutes between rounds and usually only do three to four rounds. Some days I mix it up by picking three of the exercises and doing more reps of each of them.

Jack's daily workout is very similar, but he almost always adds pullups and doubles his sets; Jack is an overachiever.

We really like this workout for the winter, because where we live in the crazy north, it's just too cold to run, wog, or walk outside. This workout takes very little time and really gets us sweating, and we feel great afterward. When we aren't doing at least little sets of exercises at least three to four times a week, our physical and mental health really seems to suffer.

DECEMBER 2017—KEEP YOUR BODY GUESSING AND DO WHAT WORKS FOR YOU:

In December I did another extended fast like the one I've already written about. But I also started to mix things up leading into it by doing black plates (keto-style) during the week, along with my intermittent or window fasting, and then carbing up on the weekend, and it worked very well for me.

I continued to see and feel benefits from my window fasts and 24-hour fasts, especially in my focus and productivity. I actually returned to this plan once the holidays were over in

January because it just works so darn well for me. I think it would work for many people too, so I wanted to share it here. I've outlined what a typical week would like below, but feel free to adjust this to make it work for you! That's what is so amazing about this lifestyle—it's totally flexible, and will fit with whatever works for you.

There is freedom here. There is grace here. There is feeling and looking so dang good!

It's all about you, and YOU CAN DO IT!

> A couple of tips before I get into the sample: don't forget to eat those healthy fats before any fast, since it really helps curb hunger. I also like to come out of a fast with a handful of nuts. Jack and I tend to eat three to four Brazil nuts per day as they are a great source of vitamins and minerals.

Below are some different options for a 6-week fasting regimen to keep things mixed up:

WEEK 1

MONDAY: WINDOW FAST 3 p.m.-10 p.m. (black plates only)
TUESDAY: 24-HOUR FAST (coffee, tea, water, and salt only)
WEDNESDAY: (black plates only)
THURSDAY: WINDOW FAST 5 p.m.-10 p.m. (black plates only)
FRIDAY: 24-HOUR FAST- (coffee, tea, water, and salt only)
SATURDAY AND SUNDAY: Gray all day—yay!

WEEK 2

MONDAY: WINDOW FAST 5 p.m.-10 p.m. (black plates only)

TUESDAY: Black plates only (keto-style)

WEDNESDAY: WINDOW FAST 5 p.m.-10 p.m. (black plates only)

THURSDAY: WINDOW FAST 5 p.m.-10 p.m. Black plates only (keto-style)

FRIDAY: 24 HOUR FAST (coffee, tea, water, and salt only)

SATURDAY AND SUNDAY: Gray all day—yay!

WEEK 3

PERIOD WEEK (A.K.A Aunt Flow is in town): (DO WHATEVER THE FRIG YOU WANT!)

WEEK 4

MONDAY: WINDOW FAST 5 p.m.-10 p.m. (black plates only)

TUESDAY AND WEDNESDAY: 48-hour FAST (water and salt only)

THURSDAY: (black plates only) 3 meals

FRIDAY: (black plates only) 3 meals

SATURDAY AND SUNDAY: gray all day—yay!

WEEK 5

AMP UP THOSE KETONES WEEK: DON'T FORGET YOUR LEAFY GREEN VEGGIES AND MAGNESIUM THIS WEEK

MONDAY: WINDOW FAST 5 p.m.-10 p.m. (black plates only)

TUESDAY: WINDOW FAST 5 p.m.-10 p.m. (black plates only)

WEDNESDAY: WINDOW FAST 5 p.m.-10 p.m. (black plates only)

THURSDAY: WINDOW FAST 5 p.m.-10 p.m. (black plates only)

FRIDAY: WINDOW FAST 5 p.m.-10 p.m. (black plates only)

SATURDAY: (black plates only) 3 meals

SUNDAY: (black plates only) 3 meals

WEEK 6

LET'S BREAK A LONG STALL* WEEK: DON'T FORGET YOUR LEAFY GREEN VEGGIES AND MAGNESIUM THIS WEEK

MONDAY: WINDOW FAST 5 p.m.-10 p.m. (black plates only)

TUESDAY: EGGS-ONLY FAST* (three times today)

WEDNESDAY: WINDOW FAST 5 p.m.-10 p.m. (black plates only)

THURSDAY: EGGS-ONLY FAST (three times today)

FRIDAY: (black plates only) 3 meals

SATURDAY AND SUNDAY (black plates only) 3 meals

*An egg-only fast is where you eat *only* eggs prepared

however you like them, but JUST eggs and cruciferous veg-etables. You can cook them in coconut or avocado oil, or in butter. And if I'm really hungry, I might even steal a piece or two of Jack's bacon.

*I consider a long stall to be more than six to eight weeks without seeing any weight loss. You can also do a two-day back-to-back "eggs-only fast" if you think you can stand two days of just eggs. This should only be used if you've tried ev-erything else, including mixing up your plates and being sure to move every day. Make sure you aren't just stuck in a rut.

Just like with my plate colors, I fast "on the fly," mean-ing that if a friend calls up and wants to meet for lunch and a glass of wine, I'm not going to pass it up because I was fasting. This is what's so great about this for me: there are no points to count; I don't have to overthink anything. I adjust my plans depending on what works best for my life on that particular day.

As a great example, Jack decided last night that he really wanted us to go hear a new musician at a local hot spot. This was a spur of the moment thing, so I changed my fasting win-dow a bit so we could have a burger on a gluten-free bun and a brew together, and we really enjoyed ourselves.

Life is short and this mama does *not* have time for count-ing macros, calculations, points, or guilt! There are days when I all I want is a burger on a gluten-free bun, and I won't de-prive myself of that. There are days when I feel like it would be pretty easy not to eat, and there's not much on the schedule, so

I just go with the flow.

Now, I know this might not work for everyone. There are people who really need to have things planned out. My work schedule is flexible, so I can take days off and work at night. Some people can't do that and I totally understand that they might need a stricter fasting and eating schedule. Jack sticks to a 16:8 window during the week because that's what works for him; a 16:8 window is where you fast for sixteen hours out of the day and eat throughout the remaining eight hours. He loves to work out while fasting and says it's easy to go as long as eighteen hours without even thinking about eating. Does that mean that he might adjust his window to open early on occasion so we can have a nice lunch date? Heck, yes!

If there's anything the past year has taught me, it's that you need to make this work not just for a season, but for a lifetime. There are so many "diets" out there, so many things that seem to work for six months, a year, maybe even two years. I follow a ton of people on social media who diet using exercise and calorie restriction, losing all the weight only to put it right back on. Unfortunately, life and biology happen, and they get stressed and eat, or have a setback and can't exercise as much, or their bodies simply adjust to 1500 calories a day, and then they're back right where they started—or, as I've experienced, with an extra twenty or fifty pounds. We've all seen this happen, right? You can't expect that life will suddenly become easy and perfect once you've lost the weight.

Over the past year I have been trying to figure out a way to keep my body and mind healthy and happy while still being able to truly live my life. This means doing all the things that really make me feel like I'm living. I don't want to sit on the sidelines watching everyone else living. I've been there, done that, and it's no fun.

Fasting gives me this freedom. If I know there's a big family event approaching and everyone is going to be partying—like this weekend when my little boy turns six—but on Friday I have a day of working and running around and nothing fun happening, it will be super easy for me to fast on Friday so I can really enjoy my weekend and still feel great while keeping my body in the best health.

This really works long-term because when we fast we actually see an increase in the speed of our metabolism. People who fast in the long term actually experience a process that is steady and easy to maintain, which is a very different experience from the eternal struggle so many chronic dieters face.

I don't know about you, but I would rather fast periodically and know my metabolism is revving up, detoxing, and healing instead of worrying about the same stubborn pounds for the millionth time in my life.

BONUS FAST (AUGUST 2017):

I sometimes wish I was able to keep things to myself, but God made me an open book, so here it goes, full disclosure. In August 2017, a couple days into a planned 5-day fast, I had my 20-year high school reunion. Who doesn't want to look good when they're about to meet people they haven't seen in twenty years? Well, I decided I would do an extended fast beforehand, because why wouldn't I want to be glowing and floating? Well, as soon as Jack and I arrived downstate where my reunion was taking place I just didn't feel like fasting anymore. I think at that point I was about twenty-four to thirty-six hours into it; I had started a bit before we actually started the drive down, and I just wanted to celebrate with him and eat.

Our hotel was right across from one the restaurants we loved to go to when we lived down there. It wasn't that I was very hungry, since I was past the peak of hunger by then, but I really just wanted the have the social experience and fun of going out to eat with my husband. I wanted to sit with him and drink wine and have a yummy chopped salad and steak. This was such a rare and special thing and I knew I shouldn't and wouldn't pass it up.

So you know what I did? I broke my fast and had dinner with my husband and I had NO regrets. So much so that even now it puts a smile on my face just thinking about it. I felt great, and everyone said I looked great.

There's so much I feel like I missed out on in life because of my health and my fears. Now, because of some recent life experiences, I've found that having a life balance sweetens the joy, which levels out the bad, worrisome, and challenging parts. Life just feels that much more vibrant to me. It's not that my life has changed, but what has changed is how I choose to experience my life.

The other interesting thing about fasting is that I've become even more picky about what I put into my body. Yes, I am a total food snob. It's amazing when you don't eat for a day, or days, how picky you'll be about what you actually decide to eat, once you're done fasting. You want only the best things. I crave things that are good for me. You couldn't pay me to put junk in my body, these days. I want the best steak, or the perfectly seasoned grilled organic chicken, or crisp green salads with creamy dressing, or all the steamed vegetables with real butter. I want cheese—the best aged cheddar—and dark, *dark*, chocolate. These are the foods of the gods! I want them all.

This hasn't been a 180-degree change for me because, as you know, I've been working on eating healthy food for some time. It's just that now I am more focused on achieving a clean-health goal. I'm really mindful about what sort of food is going into my body, focusing on which fuels make my body feel the best. I've also really worked on the practice of eating more slowly, and setting a pretty table. I want the act of eating to be an act of thanks and gratitude. I don't want to take for granted that so many people experience true hunger and have so much less, so I try to keep that in mind, and remind my kids that being able to sit down and eat together isn't a right, but a luxury.

The other added bonus of this lifestyle for Jack and I is an even lower food bill. My growing kids are picking up some of our slack, but overall our food bill continues to lower each week. I know everyone talks about healthy food costing so much more, but we've seen the opposite to be true. Costco and Aldi have amazing prices on good, healthy choices. Just be smart with what, how, where, and when you buy. As I've already said, food is everywhere we go, but a lot of it is really good and of high quality—that's the stuff you want.

I read an article which talked about how if Americans would all skip one meal a day and give that amount toward hunger, then world hunger would soon no longer exist. That might be a tad extreme, but I do think there's something very powerful in the idea. How cool would it be if people who fasted took some of that extra grocery money and gave it to organizations dedicated to eliminating world hunger? What if we could heal our own bodies at the same time as we help heal someone else? That thought brings tears to my eyes.

Our family has recently started to buy an extra bag of groceries each time we shop. We give the food to a local pantry that caters exclusively to homeless teens in our area. It was very eye-opening for us to learn that half the kids in our local high school don't have a permanent residence, so this donation really spoke to us. I suggest doing something like this if you have kids, because it has really helped my kids be mindful of wastefulness, and more aware of our daily blessings.

It's a great thing!

Some other life changes have come out of my fasting experience: an increased desire to open our home to hospitality; increased love of collecting cool cookbooks; inspired interest in exotic recipes and tasty treats.

Having these periods when you aren't eating helps you think about ways you could use the meals you'd ordinarily be eating to feed others. Totally weird, I know! I've been thinking a lot lately about how I could prepare meals for friends or neighbors who might be having a rough day. Not only has it been on my heart during this season, but my family has commented about how we could be more hospitable to our community too. In fact, after reading a book about serving our neighbors, we've decided to make it a family project.

I think our entire health journey has bonded our family around food in a very unique way. Running together, eating together, and discussions about health have created a way for us to also teach and serve others. I'm not at all saying this to brag or boast, but just to share that even with a few lazy teenagers and cranky toddlers, God has given our family some really cool experiences. If your family is crazy like mine, check out the Turquoise Table Project at www.kristinschell.com/how-does-it-work

WHAT A RANDOM FASTING DAY LOOKS LIKE:

A day in the life of a faster looks like any other person's day, but a faster has SO MUCH MORE TIME. Eating, even when you're doing other things as well, takes so much freaking *time*. Trust me when I say that on the days that I'm fasting I literally have extra HOURS in my day.

I wake up and grab my coffee, and then I spend some time

alone, unless my baby wakes up super early, which doesn't happen often but when it does it totally and completely throws me right off. But usually I get a solid half hour to myself. My amazing husband Jack leaves before dawn to take our oldest to school. It's a 45-minute drive each way for them, so half of our house is empty when I wake up, and let me tell you, silence in our home is so rare that this half hour gives me an embarrassing amount of joy. I have a special chair where I sit and journal, and I write out five to ten things I'm grateful for, and then I list five things I want to affirm to myself. Most days these are just a few words each, but there are days when I feel thankful for the chair I'm sitting in and the air in my lungs. Whatever it is, I WRITE IT OUT. Nothing is too small.

Since studying Enneagrams and learning I'm a type 4, a romantic or individualist, I know I require this solitude and this time each morning to be centered. On the days when I don't get this time, a major disturbance occurs—it messes up my whole mojo, just ask Jack!

Then I wake up the little guys and fix them something to eat. In the beginning, getting food ready for them in the morning was tough, but now it isn't really difficult at all. I honestly don't even think about food until my body tells me I need to eat. It took me getting out of my head regarding food so I could focus on my body for me to reach this point of self-awareness.

After breakfast I get them dressed—or they get themselves dressed, depending on the kid—and then Jack comes back just in time to take the little boys to school. We are very,

very lucky that the little boys' school is much closer than the older kids' school is. When Jack gets back, we have a quick workout or morning meeting, depending on what's on deck for us that day.

We usually try to warm up our muscles with a hot shower, or have some time under red lights, or jump in the hot tub or bathtub. Then we do a quick workout and usually we do a cool or cold shower. I've learned the extreme temps before and after working out are both really good for my body and, in particular, my skin. If you have access to a sauna at a gym, I highly recommend using that. Steam rooms and/or saunas are so great for your heart and overall health. Jack and I are both on team sauna! We've found most people don't take advantage of them at their health club or gym; don't be those people! If you have one you can access, we *highly* recommend getting some time in it.

Then we work. We've discovered that our most productive hours are between 10 a.m. and 2 p.m., so we try to spend those hours without any distractions, maximizing our productivity. The awesome thing about fasting is that as long as we have our salt and water, we don't stop until we have to pick up the kids in the afternoon. This works so well that if I was at a 9-5 desk job I might ask my boss if I could leave early if I worked through lunch. Jack and I have both found that when we fast, we get *so* much more done, and our focus is crazy sharp. I'm talking laser sharp, people.

Then we spend time with the kids when they get home from school, usually helping with homework or getting them ready for after-school activities. Karri usually helps me with dinner because we also have 150 animals to feed twice a day, and between that and feeding the kids things can be a bit overwhelming. I know, I know—it's a circus! We get the food prepared and then one of two things happens: the kids will sit down to dinner with Karri and Sam, or we all sit down and I have some LaCroix. If I have some social media to check, there are times I'll run back into my office while the family eats, but I try not to do that unless it's really important.

After everyone is done eating, we do a family devotional and talk about our day. Usually we go around the table and talk about the best most challenging parts of our day, or sometimes we count our blessings, and if someone has a birthday we go around saying what we love most about that person. Then we usually hang out reading in our living room, or we watch something silly that the whole family will enjoy. Some of our favorite TV shows are *THE CURSE OF OAK ISLAND*, *FIXER UPPER*, and *FULLER HOUSE*. Yes, we are a family of *dorks*!

Once we get the kids to bed, Jack and I either read together or Jack reads to me—super sappy, maybe, but he's a great reader! Or we might take a walk around the farm, sit and listen to music, or light some candles and just chill…and you know what "chill" means! If we need to laugh, we watch a comedy special on Netflix or sometimes we just go to bed early like the old people we are. LOL!

Some days, fasting just isn't going to work. The struggle is just too much and things become too stressful. When fasting becomes a curse and not a blessing, I change up my plans by opening up an eating window and then decide what will work best for me the next day. It is all about flexibility and what works.

I also have to issue an important warning about eating disorders and triggers, which might cause some unhealthy eating habits. As I said before, I think that fasting is part of the design of our body and that it's totally natural to fast. I also think it can be very good for us to fast for spiritual occasions, but—and this is a pretty big *BUT*—if you've had any issues with eating disorders or self-abuse and punishment of your body via withholding food, fasting can trigger that and you might fall back into unhealthy eating habits.

If this is the case, fasting may not be the best idea for you; as I've said elsewhere several times, if you have a specific health concern, speak to your doctor before beginning any kind of fasting regimen

Having fasting as a tool in your tool belt as you work on attaining your best health is great! It's just another way to keep your body guessing, and working on being your very best you.

Just be very careful, always stop your fast if you don't feel well, and always discuss things with your doctor, since you and your doctor are the best two people to make any and all decisions about your health.

JANUARY 2018 AND BEYOND—FASTING, EATING, LOVING, AND LIVING:

I'm not sure how many extended fasts, if any, I'll do going forward unless they are specifically dedicated to spiritual reasons. Why? Mostly because I'm not sure it's necessary for me, at this stage of my journey. I think if you have less than 25 percent body fat, fasting more than about three days per quarter really isn't necessary. I'll probably do a 3-day water fast every quarter for the anti-cancer and health benefits, as well as for cell regrowth. With my previous health issues, this makes sense as a preventative measure.

On the whole, doing 16, 18, or even 24-hour fasts are good for me during the week, but there are days when I'm super busy and want to be more productive and focused, and fasting makes it pretty easy for me. Jack often comments on how crazy it is that he doesn't even think about food most days until the afternoon.

The most important thing for us these days is making sure we're enjoying good, whole, healthy foods in a way that not only works best for our bodies but also for our lifestyle. At this point, neither of want to miss out on dinner with our kids, and both of us want as much focus and minimal distraction during the day.

For me, the longer fasts do require more brain space and I think I'll continue to do those leading up to Easter and Christmas like I did in 2017. It helped me keep my spiritual focus sharp during those seasons, and it slowed those seasons down for me, which was a welcome benefit.

Tomorrow, this could change—Jack and I are always talking about how we're feeling, and making the necessary adjustments. Usually we do this with the seasons: are we sleeping well? Are we stressed? How is our performance with our workouts? Do we have runs and training coming up that might require more carbs? All these things factor into our decision making, and these are questions we regularly ask ourselves.

Jack and I firmly believe in eating with the season. In the summer we're going to find our friends at the farmer's market and eat all of the yummy foods they grow. As I sit here writing looking out the window at the icy cold winter landscape, I can't tell you what I would do for some fresh blueberries straight from the farmer's market. If I think really hard, I can almost taste them.

In the summer and fall Jack and I tend to eat more white plates just because of the fresh, harvested fruits and vegetables we can get fresh locally. We then go into what my husband calls "KETO winter," where we tend to eat more black plates and fats like the big bears we are. This seasonal, natural way to let your body go into a more ketogenic state is really smart, economical, and great for your health long-term. We've also found this tends to make us feel warmer in the winter. #bonus

Jack and I are always reevaluating, but we really like how our bodies feel when we let nature dictate what we eat and when. I also think this aligns with how our bodies were designed and how people ate before we had convenience stores and fast food on every corner. We do have four very distinct seasons where we live, and I know it isn't the same for everyone reading this book, but I think leaning toward a natural cycle is something anyone can do no matter where you live. Ask yourself which foods are naturally available in the season where you are now? How do those foods make you feel in that season? We've found the foods that make us feel the most satisfied in those seasons are usually the foods most available to us at that moment. The great thing about eating this way is we save money and support our local farmers' economy in the process. Everyone is a winner here!

Finding what works for you takes some time and effort, but mostly it just requires some flexibility and fluidity. I know that some people find it's too hard, or that they don't have time, but once you're tuned into your body and are feeling great, your body will give you signals and let you know what you need and when you need it. I promise.

One thing that I'm constantly discussing with the women I coach is that you have to keep mixing things up and keep your body guessing. When we get into a rut it's a sign that our bodies are adapting and stalling. Whenever this happens I suggest changing the pattern of plate colors, the types of foods you're eating, and when. This usually shakes things loose.

As I look back at my own journey over the past three years, I see a gradual evolution, and periodic and/or window fasting is another tool in my toolbox. I'll use it when I need it, if I need it, and only in ways that make me feel good. I must remain conscious of my goals and my mental and physical health; I don't want to get into a trap of obsession over what

I'm eating or when. This is something that would be very easy to do, personally. In my journaling, meditation, and prayer, seeking a balance with my health always my primary focus. For much of my life I gave up so much of my headspace to eating, and food, and how I looked. Now, nearing forty, I'm striving to give that space over to something else, something better.

I've recently started doing a class that's part yoga and part meditation, and what I hope to gain is a stronger connection between my mind and body, creating peace with my mind and body, and peace with where my body was and where it's headed. I'm making friends with both the body I once had and the body I have now. I'm learning to love even those parts of me that make me cringe, the parts that aren't as secure, and the parts that honestly still hurt and are healing.

Fasting has given me a respect for my body, and for food. It might sound dramatic, but through fasting I learned that my body didn't always need to have what I thought it did, and that frequently it needed things I never even thought about. I learned how deeply my mind and body are connected. I never really understood how important this component was until I started fasting and discovered how easy it was for me to only listen to my mind, and ignore my body. And I'm still learning.

The most important thing I've learned is to never give up on your personal growth, and that we all deserve good health. Good health shouldn't just be for other people, or those with the best willpower, or the athletes. Good health is so important because it literally does change your life in a way I never understood until I had it. Now that I'm in good health, that burden is gone. That's a heavy load to carry for so many years, and I'm overjoyed to be free of it. It's worth EVERYTHING to have that freedom.

I won't ever give up my wellness journey and my lifestyle, because I finally know how freedom feels.

Common Fasting Intervals

I'M GOING TO REMIND YOU YET AGAIN HOW IMPORTANT IT is to do what works for you and your lifestyle. The beauty of this is that it's *so* flexible! Do what makes you feel good and gives you the best quality of time. Don't stress yourself out or push yourself too hard if something doesn't feel right. If you don't feel good during a fast, and water and salt doesn't help, STOP. There's always another day to try again!

> As always, discuss this with your doctor, especially if you plan on trying a longer fast and you take daily medication.

12-HOUR DAILY FAST

A standard 12-hour fast was common, until recently. Our grandparents did it and their grandparents did it, but I'm not sure they would have thought they were fasting per se. Anyone can do a 12-hour fast! Just stop eating around 8 p.m. and then eat your breakfast the next morning at 8 a.m. Easy right? Giving your body this time to rest can lower and level out your insulin. If you can space out your three daily meals evenly, you'll be in even better shape!

16–HOUR DAILY FAST:

A 16-hour fast, with an 8-hour eating window—also sometimes called the LEANGAINS method—is just a touch longer than the 12-hour fast, but it has additional health benefits if you can fit it into your lifestyle. Jack loves this interval because it seems effortless for him. For example, stop eating at 8 p.m. and then skip breakfast the next morning and fast until you eat your lunch at noon. You can also reverse this and eat breakfast and lunch and then skip dinner. We prefer to skip breakfast because dinner is such an important time for our family.

20–HOUR DAILY FAST:

A 20-hour fast with a 4-hour eating window—also sometimes called the WARRIOR or SPARTAN DIET, or sometimes OMAD (One Meal A Day, if you only eat once in that 4-hour window) is usually reserved for those in maintenance mode because the calorie-restrictive nature of it can cause some people to experience stalls. Yes, under-eating can become a problem with a short eating window. Make sure that when your window is open, you're really feasting. I also think it's a good idea with this short window not to push it too late into the evening, as that's a lot to try to eat before bed. I would recommend opening up a 4-hour window midday. I also think mixing up these various daily interval windows can be a good strategy. As I've said over and over again, it's important to keep the body guessing. Even switching your window from starting in the morning to the evening can shake things up enough to make a difference. Again, make sure whatever you choose works for your daily commitments on that particular day.

24-HOUR FAST:

A true 24-hour fast will usually go from a meal on one day to the same meal the next day. Breakfast to breakfast, lunch to lunch, or dinner to dinner. So if you had dinner at 6 p.m. today you wouldn't eat again until dinner the next day at 6 p.m. This fast works great for those who have to take daily medications or supplements, because you're able to take those each day and still fast for a full twenty-four hours. This is a nice fasting interval for me to mix into my week every so often. I prefer this over a fast with a 4-hour window. It's also easy to do if I close my window after dinner around six and then open it up the next evening and go into some solid black plates, and then do another 24-hour fast. It feels fairly easy for me, and I've found I have great energy.

The weekend before a 24-hour fast I'll have a few white plates and then switch things up the next week. I've found that the changes in eating patterns and plates are really great for my body and how I feel. Again, this is just what I think is best for me, and experimenting with different patterns and plates will make you an expert at what feels best and works best for you. Take the time and really listen to your body, and once you have the hang of it you'll be operating in superhuman mode. You'll be feeling so good that you might even want to wear a cape! This doesn't happen overnight, but I promise you'll get there. Keep it up!

FASTING EVERY OTHER DAY:

With this fasting protocol you would fast every other day; for example eat on Monday, fast Tuesday, eat on Wednesday, fast Thursday, eat Friday, fast Saturday, and eat Sunday. I think this ends up being tricky for most people, so it isn't one of my favorite fasts to recommend. If this works well for your lifestyle then absolutely try it, but remember that if you're taking daily medication this can be hard especially if you happen to miss a day. Please make sure to talk to your health provider if this is something you decide you want to try. Also important to remember is that on eating days you really need to feast to keep your metabolism moving.

36-HOUR FAST:

This fast is one of my favorites, because it seems to go pretty easily for me since I'm sleeping for a pretty big chunk of it. If you plan it just right, you reach peak hunger—usually around hour 18—when you're sleeping, and that little trick makes this one much easier. So, if you finish your dinner at about 6 p.m. Monday, you would totally skip eating Tuesday and then eat breakfast on the third day, Wednesday. This means I only miss eating dinner with my kids on one evening, but I'm getting in a full thirty-six hours of fasting. Usually I'll feel so amazing by the third day that I can usually even go a bit longer, and most times I'm pretty close to hitting that 48-hour mark if I feel really great. This is probably my second-favorite fasting interval. It's a bit tricky at first, because the 18- to 24-hour mark can be hard, but once you have a good handle on it, this can be a fairly easy fasting interval for most people. The biggest issue I have with this fasting interval is remembering to take my medicine on eating days. I fixed that by setting daily reminders on my phone so I wouldn't forget.

What did we do before smartphones?

42-HOUR FAST:

I actually do this one pretty frequently, because when I go for a 36-hour fast I often just keep it going until I'm at forty-two hours. I don't think I've ever set out to do a 42-hour—it just happens naturally. An example of this would be, as I said above, starting a fast at 6 p.m. and then not eating at all on day two, and then breaking your fast at lunch on the third day. This is probably more common for me than the 24-hour fast because I usually feel best with just coffee for breakfast.

EXTENDED FAST: (ANYTHING OVER FORTY-EIGHT HOURS)

Of all the extended fasts I've done, my absolute favorite is the three-day. I feel great after I finish it, and there are really no adverse side effects. I would caution that doing any extended fasts in the three- to five-day range is something you really should build up to. Fasting is a muscle like any other, so you have to make it stronger through constant exercise. If you jump into an extended fast right away, you run the risk of burning out, not feeling well, or you don't see the results you thought you would.

Please take my advice and make sure you've prepared your body and mind before you attempt an extended fast. Make sure you have lots of water, you've eaten some fatty meals beforehand so you aren't in carb-crave mode, you're well rested, and you don't have stressful meetings or other big life events happening during your planned fast.

And, as always, if at any time you aren't feeling well, and water and salt isn't helping, STOP YOUR FAST!

It's important to recognize that most people gain back

about half of the weight they lost during a fast because most of that is water weight. Don't worry though, because numbers aren't what this is about. Most of the benefits I've had from fasting are in my body composition, which is something most people begin to see almost instantly. I encourage you to take photos of your face and body throughout the process so you can see your progress with skin condition, overall appearance, and any trouble spots you might have. For example, Jack had lots of fat in his abdominal area that showed remarkable changes almost instantly.

Three cheers for melting that visceral fat away!!!

Jack also does lots of physical activity while fasting, usually doing both heavy lifting and CrossFit-type workouts. He's seen major changes in his muscles—which proves you won't lose muscle mass from fasting. We've seen the reverse to be true.

As a final note, remember to keep up with your salt on an extended fast; I always load up on my electrolytes prior to attempting an extended fast.

> Important note: there is a medical complication that can arise from doing a long extended fast, called "re-feeding syndrome." It's usually seen in people who are already malnourished and have been fasting and then return to eating after a long amount of time. Although very uncommon, it can happen and this is one of the reasons why I caution that anyone attempting longer extended fast (over five days) needs to be under the care and monitoring of a doctor.

WHEN FASTING DON'T FORGET:

- S.O.S.: suck on salt. Salt is your fasting friend and will keep your electrolytes in balance.
- WATER, WATER, WATER: make sure you have water on hand. I personally won't even attempt any sort of fast past twelve hours without an entire case of plain LaCroix at the ready. There is an app called Water-minder, which reminds you to drink water every hour, if you need help remembering to drink consistently.
- You *can* still work out. One of the ways we stay busy and keep our minds off food is by moving. I love to do yoga, walk, or some stretching followed by a salt bath in the evenings of my fasting days.
- If you aren't going for autophagy, don't forget you can still enjoy coffee or tea with your fasts. I've also done a bit of bone broth on occasion during some of my extended fasts. I've also been known to have some pickles or pickle juice, as those seem to help me over the rough spots, too.
- Hunger *does* peak, and it *will* get better! Just hold on and I promise, if you're sticking to your water and salt and you try to "ride the wave" of your hunger, it *will* go away.

Three Fasting Success Stories

WHEN I WRITE THESE BOOKS, I OFTEN REACH OUT TO friends and family to see if anyone is willing to be my guinea pigs and try some of my advice or techniques. Isn't that nice of me? So I wanted to share three awesome stories from friends who will remain anonymous.

The first is a forty-year-old male friend who is in pretty good shape except for his midsection—very similar to Jack. He works out often and, except for his tummy, you'd probably say he was athletic in build. He never had issues with weight growing up, but as he's aged you can see his midsection getting larger each year. He recently cut out sugar and is lowering his carbohydrate intake in the hopes of reducing his midsection.

The reason extra midsection weight is so scary is that there's a direct correlation between it and heart health. Men who carry weight there often have a lot of visceral fat, which can't be seen. I suggested this friend try skipping lunch and trying for a daily 16:8 fast. In only a month we saw some positive changes to his waist measurements. This was without *any* other dietary changes. Full disclosure: he was even having some cheat meals and beer on the weekends. He told me this fasting regimen seems very maintainable for him, and he doesn't miss his breakfast toast at all.

The second is a twenty-five-year-old female friend. She has always struggled with her weight and has tried everything to get rid of what she would call her "muffin top." She recently lost about twenty pounds; she is very petite, and all of her excess weight is around her midsection. She eats clean and is physically active, and is currently at a normal BMI, but her muffin top area still bothers her because she hasn't had children yet and she's worried about having extra weight in that area before trying to conceive.

We again started with a 16:8 interval window, and then went to a 5-hour window fast on occasion to mix things up. She also did various plate combinations as she also follows my plan daily, and feels best having carbs in the evening. She eventually decided she would do 5-hour windows during the week alternating white and black plates during her eating windows, and then doing longer windows on the weekend, usually a 16:8. Within just a few weeks we were seeing results. She stuck to this plan of window fasting with alternating plates for a few weeks, and then went back to longer widows with great success. Although her progress is slower than my male friend—don't those men just always have it easier?—she is really happy and she feels really good eating this way, and doesn't feel deprived at all. She also told me that her sleeping and focus have both improved since experimenting with fasting.

The third story is from a sixty-year-old female. This friend has been doing my program, and she's lost about forty pounds. She had about ten more to go and was looking to change things up so she could get those last few pounds off. Her doctor suggested she increase her exercise, but honestly she wasn't sure how she would do that as she was already walking/wogging at least four to five days a week. After doing a few weeks of window or intermittent fasting at various intervals, she decided to try one or two 24-hour fasts each week. After doing this for only a few weeks, those pounds were *gone*!

We both couldn't believe how quickly she reached her goal. I think the most important thing here was that she stayed active; she continued walking, fasted clean, and feasted when it was time to eat. I was so proud of her! The other great thing about this is that she also commented on how easily these adjustments were for her. It was a bit tricky at the start simply because she had been eating breakfast right when she woke up for so many years, but once she got the hang of window fasting, the 24-hour fasts weren't much harder. She eased into it. She's continuing to mix up her fasting intervals with whatever works for her at the time, and she is easily maintaining her weight loss.

Don't Fast from Sexy Times!

(AND OTHER IMPORTANT TIPS FROM JACK)

Y WIFE HAS WRITTEN A LOT SO FAR ABOUT ALL THE different ways you can fast, and all the different things you can fast from. It's a lot to take in, am I right? 24-hour fasts, 36-hour fasts, window fasting, extended fasts; fasts from food, fasts from social media, fasts from negativity, and fasts from mindless consumerism.

You know what you absolutely should NOT fast from? SEX.

Yeah, yeah, I'm a guy, so of course I'm going to say this. But you know what? Jasinda agrees. I mean, she's letting *me* write a chapter about it, so you know she's serious.

I'm sure you all know the facts about the benefits of sex, but I'll go over them anyway, just to be sure we're all the same page.

First of all, sex has the capacity to make you happier. I'm

not saying it WILL, just that it CAN—sex releases both oxy-tocin and dopamine, among other fun neurochemicals. If you want the detailed science, just Google "What happens to the brain during sex?" and have fun with the search results. My point is, a bad day can be made better by engaging in some quality naked snuggles with your partner. It's not going to fix any problems, obviously, but when you can escape for a few minutes and end up feeling better, lighter, and happier, you'll end up with a renewed ability to deal with the sucky things that happen in life.

Second, sex is exercise, which means it burns calories. Ready for some fun facts? Men burn on average 100 calories in an average sexual encounter, and women 69—my wife would kill me if I made a crude joke about that second number, so I'm going to refrain. Now, obviously, the number of calories burned varies depending on how long you have sex for and how...erm...vigorous you are. So ladies, if your husband is resistant to the idea of exercise or running, get him in bed and make him sweat! You're helping him burn calories while engaging happy hormones in each other's brains! Everybody wins!

Since I'm talking about burning calories, let's compare sex to running, shall we? Running is great exercise, let's be clear. It burns calories, helping you shed pounds and inches, makes your heart and lungs stronger, and puts you in overall better shape, reducing your risk of less than awesome things like heart disease. Assuming you're following my wife's advice regarding proper healthy nutrition—which, since you're reading this, I'm assuming you're at least interested in getting healthier—my point is this: if a man runs a kilometer, he burns around 105 calories, and women burns 91; if you walk a kilometer, men burn 52 calories, and women 43. If a 150 lb person runs five kilometers—3.1 miles—at a 10-minute per mile pace, he or she would burn around 230 calories. Obviously, the faster you run, the more you burn. So you can have sex and burn 100 calories, or you can run a kilometer and burn 100 calories. I'm just saying—only one of those activities releases dopamine and oxytocin.

I'm not saying sex should be your ONLY exercise, just that it DOES count, and if you're hesitant to try running or lifting weights, but you still want to get more physically active, you could consider getting "active" with hubby tonight, and see how much sweat you can work up in the process. He'll thank you, and your bodies and minds and metabolisms will thank you, too.

Bonus prizes if you have vigorous, sweaty, crazy monkey sex while fasting, because when you're fasting, your body is already burning fat, and when you work out, you ramp up your metabolism, meaning, you'll start burning MORE calories in less time, and your metabolism will CONTINUE to burn hotter for a while afterward as well. So, fasted sex means more calories burned. Even more winning!

I suppose I should talk about fasting on its own, huh? Listen, I'll be honest, when my wife first talked about fasting, I was VERY skeptical. Fasting, to me, was something holy dudes in the Bible did, because they were super holy. Who would voluntarily NOT eat for a day or two or three just because it was "healthy"? Crazy talk.

I know my wife isn't crazy, or if she is, she's crazy like a fox. I can't even tell you how many times she's said to me, *"Jack, I know you're gonna think I'm crazy, but I want to try something…"* which usually means I'm going to end up trying it too. That's how this whole health journey started; Jasinda said to me, *"Jack, I know you're gonna think I'm crazy, but I want to try and cut out refined carbs and sugar, and see if it'll help me feel better. And…I think you should do it with me."* I hated the idea, especially when she explained all the foods that fell under the umbrella of refined carbs and sugar. But I trust my wife, because she's so much smarter than I am in so many ways, so I tried it. And I felt better. I stopped getting the shakes, stopped crashing midday, stopped having energy spikes and crashes, and the soft, doughy pillow of fat around my midsection started to disappear.

I had more energy as a result, which meant I finally, for the first time in my entire life, found the motivation to start working out regularly. At first, it was just to help accelerate the rate at which the pudge in my middle went away, but then I found myself genuinely enjoying throwing around kettlebells and finishing 5K races.

Bear with me, I WILL get around to fasting, eventually.

As we continued our journey to health, we played around with lots of things—carbs only in the morning, carbs only at night, carb cycling every other day, carbs only on the weekends, no carbs at all for certain periods of time. We played with the kinds of carbs, and how much we consumed at a time.

More veggies, more protein. More healthy fats.

Yes, Jack, beer is a carb. Even the low-carb kind.

The more I committed to getting healthy, the more I enjoyed it. Once I detoxed from refined carbs—meaning, primarily, Cheez-Its and pizza and French fries—I found my tastes changing. If you read the chapter I wrote about veggies, this is familiar territory to you. The process of changing taste buds continues for me, even to this day. I'll never eat lima beans, *ever*, but I *have* discovered that I actually enjoy asparagus, especially if it's cooked in lots of butter and garlic and the tips are all crispy. I like broccoli just fine, but it turns me into a walking fart cannon, so I have to limit how much of it I eat for the sake of the environment and my family's olfactory sanity. I like onions. I LOVE avocado. I eat a huge baby spinach salad every day, usually with lots of cheese and bacon bits and avocado.

Chicken and turkey strips still do NOT count as bacon, though.

I got more into lifting weights. We started using the sauna—doing pushups and planks and squats in the sauna is, it turns out, crazy intense and insanely effective.

And then, one day, my wife said those perilous words, which usually end up changing my life somehow: *"So, Jack. I want to try something, and you're probably going to think I'm crazy."* And she started talking about this book she'd read which promoted fasting as the fastest and most effective way of losing fat. We started listening to podcasts about fasting, and she would tell me about all the books she'd read, and the facts and statistics on how great fasting is for so many reasons. And then, one day, she said she was going to try it. She was going to fast. I was like, you go, girl—I'll be over here eating breakfast LIKE A NORMAL PERSON.

Joke's on me.

She skipped breakfast, and didn't pass out. Okay, well… I've skipped breakfast and been fine, so sure, skipping breakfast can't be all THAT hard, right? And then she skipped breakfast AND lunch. She was a little cranky midday, but she ate some salt and drank a lot of water and locked herself in her office, and ate dinner with us and was fine. Then she realized she'd eaten carbs the night before she fasted, and decided to try eating a black plate the night before instead (full honesty, here? I still get black and white plates mixed up, and I'm married to her, so if you still need a cheat sheet, don't feel too bad!). The next time she decided to try a fast, she had a big omelet and bacon for dinner while the rest of us had whatever our dinner was. She skipped breakfast and lunch the following day…and didn't get as hangry midday. Dinnertime came around, and she claimed she felt amazing and was going to try to skip dinner too and see how she felt. She ended up doing some work while we ate dinner that night, and then we all spent the evening watching a favorite show together. It was a little weird at first, her not eating dinner with us, but then we just kind of forgot about it. She ended up going all the way to lunch the following day before she broke her fast—that was her first 36-hour fast.

She didn't die, or pass out. She didn't turn into a hangry rage-beast. She even said, the morning before she ate lunch with me—when she would have been about thirty-some hours into her fast—that she felt so good she could even work out. She didn't, not wanting to push herself too far too fast, but she felt like she could've. And, the next time she fasted, she did work out. I hovered around her like an overbearing asshole while she did jump squats and pushups and bench dips, until she told me in no uncertain terms that she felt fine and to back off.

I still wasn't convinced fasting was a great idea. And then she told me she'd lost something like fifteen pounds through fasting that month, which would have ordinarily taken her twice that amount of time just through nutrition and exercise.

She finally convinced me to try it.

Just skip breakfast, she said.

Okay, fine. Grrrr. Grumble grumble grumble.

It wasn't so bad. I ate a big lunch and felt fine.

Now skip breakfast and lunch, she told me. So I did, and I was a little hungry, but I got through it, and ate a big dinner.

Finally, she told me to try a 24-hour fast—from dinner Monday night to dinner Tuesday. I was, to be totally up front, kind of scared. All growing up, I'd known my dad was hypoglycemic, which meant he had to eat at regular intervals or he'd get shaky, and too much sugar made him feel crummy. I'd known I had it for years myself, with the same symptoms. If I went too long without eating, I'd get shaky hands. I was sure I'd get shaky, or even pass out. Jasinda had me eat an omelet and lots of bacon for dinner the previous night, and then I woke up and just had coffee and went about my day...expecting the shakes any minute. They never came. I got hungry an hour or two after I normally would have had lunch, and she told me to—can you guess? Suck on salt, and drink some bubbly water. I got really, really hungry, and started to resent the whole stupid experiment. But, I placed my trust in her. I ate some salt, drank about three cans of Pure LaCroix, and after a while, the feeling of hunger actually went away.

I remembered, then, all the years I'd spent in food service. I used to work a lot of double shifts; for the uninitiated, a double shift at a bar or restaurant means you work from open to close, usually around 9 or 10 a.m. to 9 or 10 p.m. It's a LONG day, and if it's busy there's not always time for a meal break between shifts, which often means working the whole twelve-plus hours without a real meal. I remembered all the times I'd pulled doubles without lunch or dinner, and how the feeling of hunger eventually went away, especially if we got slammed. I'd work like a madman, and the shift would end, and I'd eat and be fine. And this was working at a restaurant, *making and serving food*. You know how hard it is to run tray after tray of delicious-looking-and-smelling food for twelve hours when you haven't eaten all day? Even worse was cooking the food—the temptation to make a little extra and shove it into my mouth when no one was looking was a constant devil on my shoulder. I rarely gave in, mostly because that's a good way to lose your job on the line in a kitchen.

I realized, as I thought about all of this, that I'd actually had a lot of practice going without a meal or two, and that when I wasn't eating healthy, I rarely got the shakes, and I never passed out.

This doesn't mean fasting was suddenly easy, mind you. Fasting beyond sixteen to eighteen hours is still a challenge for me. I've done a few 3-day fasts, and those are still pretty hard for me. Not as hard as I'd imagined them to be, and they *do* get easier after the 18-hour mark. These longer fasts usually happen for me when we're traveling, because it's honestly just so much easier to travel when you don't have to worry about finding something to eat near an airport, in an airport, or eating airplane food.

What I've learned is that fasting is easier and more natural than I thought it would be. I never eat breakfast, now. I just don't want it, and feel better without it. It is completely natural to me now to just live my life in a 16:8 window. I get more done, I feel better, and it helps me stay lean.

Part of this process of discovery was learning how much visceral fat I had. Even after a few years of healthy eating and regular exercise—during which time I lost about twenty pounds—a DEXA scan revealed I was still at the upper end of the normal BMI range for an adult male of my age and height, and that my body fat was at least 3-5 percent higher than I'd thought it was. I'm not trying to look like The Rock or anything, but that was a shock to me. That information—that my BMI and body fat were so much higher than I'd thought, even after all I'd accomplished—was an impetus to start fasting. Especially because a lot of that extra fat wasn't visible—my belly is gone, now. I don't have visible abs—so no, none of those ripped beefcakes on our fiction covers are me! But the soft, doughy, Pillsbury doughboy belly I once had is pretty much gone entirely, and was when I had that DEXA scan done.

I still felt great about my progress, but I knew I wanted to and COULD do better. I wanted to add lean muscle, lose fat, and maybe even someday reveal those abs. What guy doesn't want that? More than anything, though, I knew I had to get rid of visceral fat—which is fat that's not just on your belly or butt or chest or wherever, but inside, around your organs, where no amount of proper nutrition and no amount of crunches or kettlebell swings will reach. You can only really get that visceral fat to go away by fasting, by forcing the body to use those reserves of fat for fuel.

I'd advise you to do your own research on visceral fat, where it comes from, and the risks that come with having too much of it. Basically, if a person is overweight, that person WILL have too much visceral fat; and guess what? Even after you've gone down however many sizes, lost that weight, gotten to where you want to be, you'll still have some visceral fat left inside you, because it's the hardest to get rid of. Simply put, it's the last thing to go because it can really only be reached through fasting. This doesn't mean you have to jump in and start doing a 3-day fast every week or month.

So these are the things that I discovered were true of me and for me, and why I decided to start fasting.

Along the way, I discovered I simply feel better on a daily

basis if I give my body a good fourteen to eighteen hours to really digest all the food I ate the day before, if I'm giving my body that time to rest from the exhausting work of digestion. I've also discovered that if I stop eating at 10 p.m. every night, when I wake up at 5:30 a.m., I've already fasted for eight hours. By the time I'm done getting all the kids to school, feeding the animals, and get into my office, I've only got between three and six hours of fasting left before I get to eat. And when I eat…I FEAST. I work out a lot, having found out how much I enjoy pushing my body to become stronger and faster and fitter, so I eat a *lot*, giving my body the fuel it needs to build muscle and replace the stores of energy I used.

My first step, like yours, was to cut out the junk—sugar and refined carbs. The second step was to learn how to eat more healthily, and to enjoy those healthy foods. The third step was to add fasting to my daily, weekly, and monthly life—I do a 3-day fast at least once a quarter to reset my immunity, and to really focus in on the spiritual components of my life.

The results from all this?

I'm in *far* better shape now, at thirty-six years old, than I was at eighteen or twenty-five. I can lift more, run farther and faster, I have more endurance, more power, and more willpower. I know, from all this, that I'll live longer, and be healthier as I age. I'll be around longer for my kids. I can keep up with my fourteen-year-old son, who is turning into a heck of an athlete and, I like to think, still show him a thing or two.

It's not a quick fix.

It's not an immediate process.

I didn't get this way overnight, or even in a single year.

I still have a long way to go, and a lot to learn.

Because this path to health, like everything else in life, is a journey wherein you never stop learning, and you never stop progressing.

Also, sex!

Biohacking

(AND OTHER STORIES FROM THE WILDER SIDE)

So. LET'S CHAT ABOUT SOME BIOHACKING EXPERIMENTS I did, and what the results were.

What is biohacking? Glad you asked! Biohacking is using your biology to "hack" your body's own systems.

When I first happened upon an online biohacking community, I found the things people were talking about were very thought-provoking, and I totally loved it. People were coming together to share their experiments and data about how they had made nutritional modifications to their lives to create awesome results. This is important, because what we put into our bodies totally changes the way we feel.

There are so many cool things I've learned from this new biohacking community that I want to share them with you. Many of the things they're experimenting with are not really new ideas—they are simply returning to the practices we used to use in the first place.

> Gradually work on trying these new therapies, and don't overdo it.

So, here we go. A list of biohacks for you to consider:

BIOHACK: COLD AND HEAT THERAPY

First, our bodies were designed to experience some discomfort in terms of both heat and cold. But today, for the most part, we live and work in environments strictly controlled to moderate temperatures so we don't have to experience those extremes. Most of us never get too far above or below those average temperatures unless we live in extreme environments. Our ancestors didn't have air conditioning or central heating. They would sweat; they felt the heat of the summer and they worked in that heat.

Where we live in Michigan, a mere hundred years ago we would not only feel the serious heat of summer, but also the frigid subzero temperatures of winter. Jack and I often think about having to take care of our farm without the kind of technology we have now—modern pipes fill an automatic watering system for the equines, lights help the fowl on darker days to extend egg laying, and we have shelters for the pigs and bunnies. I can't imagine feeding these animals without our modern comforts and outdoor coverings! We wear gear that makes it bearable to go out to feed our animals twice a day even when the temps get to negative numbers, which happens frequently in the winter.

Before the advent of modern technology the response of people's bodies to the cold temperatures would be so much different than mine is when I'm all bundled up to go outside, only to return to a house perfectly maintained at a comfortable seventy-three degrees.

When we think about how quickly these technological improvements have taken place in our lives, along with new chemicals being introduced and other environmental changes, it isn't hard to see how our body's complicated systems might not be able to catch up and adapt as quickly as we would like them to.

Several seasoned "biohackers" are regularly stressing their bodies by spending time in cryo-chambers. Essentially, a cryo-chamber allows you to spend a brief amount of time in extremely cold temperatures. Some recent studies have shown the benefits cold therapy has on pain relief, weight loss, reduction of inflammation, reduced cellulite, prevention of cancer and dementia, improved skin condition, treating headaches, managing anxiety and depression. Sound too good to be true?

I recently tried this, and I've got to say it's pretty interesting. Nanny Karri and I drove several hours to a Cryo Spa, where we spent about three minutes in a tube filled with freezing nitrogen. I did level two of three progressive levels, since I have done cold therapy before. The temperature in my chamber was minus 148 degrees Fahrenheit. Karri started at level one, which tops out at about minus 130 degrees. The exposure to extreme temps like this shocks the body and will not only promote new cell growth, but it also helps to start a process that will change any "white" visceral fat, that is hard to get rid of, to beige or brown fat which the body can shed more easily.

We both felt awesome after our sessions. It's hard to explain, but it wasn't the same type of cold you normally experience when it's cold outside; it's the sort of cold that almost has a burning feeling. I think the sensation was similar to running a long distance, or maybe even a sort of adrenaline/euphoria kind of feeling. It was pretty "cool." See what I did there? The session cost about thirty dollars, and because the location is pretty far from where we live unfortunately I probably won't be doing it very often. But if you want to try this, and you don't have access to a Cryo Spa, there are easy ways you can experience similar cold therapy "body hacking" tricks at home yourself.

Below is a list of a few things Jack and I do, whenever we can, to shock our bodies and help promote healthy cell growth and proper function.

- Take a cold shower. No, this isn't fun, but it is effective. If you can't go for the whole shower, then try to go as cold as you can at the very end.
- Cold bath (ice bath): also not the most fun in the world, but it will really invigorate you.
- Get a small bucket or tub and soak your feet in cold or ice water as long as you can.
- Take a short, brisk walk outside in cold weather without being totally bundled up from head to toe.
- Take a quick dip the lake. This is Jack's and my absolute favorite thing to do when the temps are cooler. Good old natural, cold lake water will really rev you up.

The opposite of exposing yourself to periods of cold is, obviously, exposure to heat. Jack and I try to do this every week. We get into a hot tub or sauna, or take a hot "lobster bath" to really get things heated up! It's even better if you can get really hot and then cool off right after. Jack and I are known to take a really hot shower and then run outside in the backyard when it is snowing outside. At night, we might even do this naked—please don't tell the neighbors! But, this is *awesome* for your body. If you want to feel really alive, try this yourself! Every single time I've done either heat or cold therapy, I end up feeling SO DARN GOOD! I'm just ready to take on the world!

I find this therapy especially effective if I'm feeling sluggish or yucky. It's especially effective, if I feel a cold coming on, to take a really hot bath to help push out some of those germs and release the toxins.

Another biohack Jack and I have been experimenting with, related to exposure to heat and cold, is working out under hot and cold conditions. This means that sometimes we might do a quick plank in the sauna, or run outside in the cold. I, especially, have seen some serious changes with my upper body from doing this a few times a week. I think of it as my own personal version of hot yoga. I just have to make sure I keep my electrolytes up, because this really makes me sweat. Again, listening to your body and understanding the difference between being challenged and uncomfortable versus hurting yourself is key.

BIOHACK: RED LIGHT THERAPY

Another biohacker method I often hear about is red light therapy. As I mentioned before, using red lights (the fancy scientific term is "photobiomodulation") has been shown to help with skin and scars as well as increasing energy. I've been experimenting with this a bit, as well.

I will tell you that some people are *really* into this, and they install special systems in their houses that are pretty darn expensive. I'm a pretty frugal mama; so I haven't been impressed enough yet to fully invest in these fancier and more elaborate systems. We did buy some basic infrared lightbulbs from Amazon; for the reasonable cost of twenty dollars it was worth it to us to give them a try. I'm not really sure how much improvement we've seen, but I think it has been worth the minimal amount of effort.

BIOHACK: GETTING ENOUGH SLEEP

Jack and I also continually work on improving our sleep. **SLEEP IS SO IMPORTANT!** If you aren't sleeping well, everything else in your life will be affected. We've tried almost everything out there: blue blocking, weighted blankets, cooling pads, magnesium, lavender, salt lamps, temperature, sex!

Out of all the things we've tried, below is a list of a few things I recommend:

- If you often work at a computer, I highly recommend getting some blue-light-blocking glasses. Several of my kids starting having sleep issues after they changed schools and were on iPads for hours during the day. Now, half of our kids wear blue glasses for school and when doing homework in the afternoon. We've seen the glasses make a big difference, especially with my teenage daughter who seemed to be the most sleep deprived.

- We all take our magnesium and minerals before bed. There are two brands that I swear by: the one I take that has added vitamins and minerals and is called Mary's Organic Night Time. Yes, this one is a bit pricey, but if you aren't sleeping well it's well worth the cost. The other I recommend that's a bit cheaper is Natural Calm. It's rare that one of these won't help you get a good night's sleep. I recommend you take it about an hour or so before you want to sleep. They're both sweetened with Stevia so don't worry about sugar spikes before bed.

- Weighted blankets: This is something we've used for years with our son who is on the autism spectrum. I recently started using one myself because it seemed to help me sleep, specifically when I was fasting. Previously, I mentioned that fasting makes you feel really "light," and when I was sleeping I think I was experiencing this lightness and it caused my body to flop around like a fish, which also caused Jack to lose his mind (he's a pretty light sleeper). So for my birthday he got me a weighted blanket that is *so* freaking soft. I absolutely fell in love with it. For Christmas we got all the kids weighted blankets, and although it cost a pretty penny we've all slept better ever since, so it was well worth the investment. We found a shop on Etsy that custom made them with our kids' favorite sports, characters, and colors, and now they are one of their favorite things. My oldest son's even glows in the dark!

- Temperature: Our bedroom is set to fifty-five degrees. I know, I know—it's chilly! But this has really helped us to get a good night's sleep. You don't have to have your bedroom as cold as we do, but I think experimenting with a lower temp than your usual comfort threshold is worth it. Warning: having it a bit colder in your bedroom may encourage you to make your own heat. Jack especially recommends this one.

- Mouth Tape: Okay, so this is something Jack is experimenting with. Using mouth tape can help promote deeper sleep. It forces you to breathe through your nose during sleep, which helps with blood oxygenation, resulting in less snoring and more rest. They're pretty cheap and worth a try if you struggle with staying asleep at night, or getting into a deep sleep.

- Early to bed and early to rise! Our family tries to take our cues from what's going on outside, just like our chickens. Did you know that chickens put themselves to bed along with the setting sun? Paying attention to our internal clock means going to bed earlier in the winter when the sun is setting. I think it's a great thing. It also helps us get up early in the morning so we can take time for journaling and getting ready for the day. This means we might miss the episode of *REAL HOUSEWIVES* everyone is talking about on Facebook the next day, but we've learned to be okay with it—it's what HULU and SLING are for! You can always enjoy those things later, and your body will thank you.

BIOHACK: FASTING

Some people would place intermittent or window fasting in the biohacking category too, so I want to at least mention it here. From my perspective, window fasting is really just eating the way humans ate before the "food revolution" sold us on the idea that to be healthy we need to eat *all the time*. If we look into the roots of the word "breakfast" it literally meant the meal you broke your fast with.

These days, not eating for eight hours seems like a fast to most of us. However, this simply isn't how our ancestors ate. When your body gets used to fasting, it will really begin to feel natural.

Some people might say adding MCT oil to coffee is a "biohack" too, so I'll add it here, but I don't really consider it a bio-hack. When I drink coffee I usually add some MCT oil to it. I've found this not only helps with burning fat and nutrient absorption, but it also seems to help me keep things "regular" if you know what I mean.

I'll talk later about some of the other supplements that are beneficial, but many in the biohacking community drink bulletproof coffee, which means adding butter to your coffee. Personally, I don't recommend this. Sure, add it to your veggies with some garlic, or fry your eggs in it, but I don't really think you need to add it to your coffee—there's just not enough evidence to convince me that this is beneficial, and good butter is expensive! I'll fix my coffee with a splash of heavy whipping cream or MCT on occasion, but you can't convince me I need the butter, too.

BIOHACK: GROUNDING A.K.A. EARTHING

Grounding or "earthing" is another hot and controversial topic on many of the biohacking forums, and it's a bit weird so we don't go all out with it as some do, but we have tried to remove our shoes whenever possible and get closer to the earth.

If you have no idea what I am talking about, the term grounding simply means having physical contact with the earth. Many people claim doing this regularly provides amazing health benefits. Now, the research is conflicted on this, so I can't say for sure that this has made a huge difference to me, but because there *is* some evidence that it could improve sleep, help with inflammation and adrenal health, increase energy, lower stress and tension, provide relief from headaches, regulate hormones, and countless other possible benefits, I think it's worth mentioning here.

The simple fact is that taking off your shoes and going for a walk is really easy to do! There are things like grounding shoes, sheets, and mats for people who strongly believe in this biohack, but I think you can just take a walk around your backyard with your shoes off, or take a walk on the beach. The effort is minimal, and the cost negligent, so it might be worth trying. Again this isn't something I'm 100 percent sold on, but I'm in the camp that if it could help me even a little bit, and all I have to do is get my feet dirty, then why not? I'm in! I'll try just about anything once and I have seen my health continue to improve by incorporating other seemingly simple things, so why not give this a whirl? Just don't get mad at me if you step on something—be careful out there!

BIOHACK: TAKE A VACATION

Here's another wild biohack for you: TAKE A VACATION! I'm speaking to myself here, too. I rarely, if ever, take a vacation and I really want to make 2018 the year when I take a break. I watched a documentary by Michael Moore that said much of Europe takes six weeks of paid vacation every year. SIX WEEKS! Can you even believe that? I can't. Most Americans get *maybe* one paid week of vacation a year.

Jack and I have taken the kids for a vacation once in the past five years. It's not easy to take the whole group anywhere, but this is something I think we really need to do. Did you know that taking a vacation can not only improve your health, but also extend your life? Especially if you can take a vacation where there's some nice sun exposure.

Yes, I know—money is tight, and yes, I know, it's hard to find the time, and, yes I know you have to plan ahead, and, yes, life and work is stressful and it's difficult to take time off, but you only live one life, and the best thing you can ever do is give your kids *you*. Memories with you, time with you, experiences with you.

Maybe you can't afford to go anywhere, but you could take a week off work and spend time doing things together as a family. Visit a local pool or beach, have a family movie day, take a hike, or go for a walk in a park, have a baking day, or make homemade ice cream and have friends over. Even if you don't leave home, the time off spent relaxing and enjoying yourself with your family will do wonders for you. Let's make a promise that we'll make this a priority together, that we'll do this for ourselves and make some seriously awesome vacation memories. I know we can do it!

BIOHACK: EATING SEASONALLY

Eating seasonally is another thing some people might call a hack, but I just think is smart and logical. First, as I've said in other books, it saves money. When you eat in season and you support your local farmers, you're doing so many good things. I know it does take some time to get to the farmers market and to do the research about farms in your area, but once you've gone, you'll wonder why you never went before. If you have a co-op close by, they are another great way to buy local when fruit and veggies are in season. When you have veggies and berries fresh from the farm, the store-bought ones just won't taste the same. I like my greens with just a tiny bit of dirt still on them—that dirt is good for you! The greens at the store have been washed over and over again with things like bleach and other chemicals.

When we eat this way we naturally fall into seasonal eating; and we end up eating fewer carbohydrates during the winter months and more in the summer because there are just more of them available and in season.

Some experts even think it's a good idea to take a look at the foods that were eaten in a particular season by your ancestors. I can't say I've gone that far, but I do think that examining what we're eating, when, and why is a good thing. Jack says he's "saving his carbs for sun and summer." I think it helps keep a steady balance in life, but I have to admit that if you have delicious fruit all year round, I'm jealous.

BIOHACKS: A SUMMARY

Over the past few years of incorporating these "hacks," Jack and I have seen some awesome changes to our overall health. It can be hard sometimes to pinpoint exactly what's working best, but I know when I look at the overall big, picture of our health, all of these things are making positive changes in the way we feel and our quality of life.

My biggest word of caution is don't overwhelm yourself by going "all in" with everything at once. We've continued to get healthier, stronger, and look younger because we've implemented these changes gradually over the past three to four years.

I sometimes imagine someone reading all of these books back-to-back and being overwhelmed by all the changes they have to make in their lives to get healthy. Please hear me when I say I you do *NOT* need to do everything at once. I actually believe the opposite is true—this process *should* be gradual.

If even one of the items on the list of biohacks seems like something you could do, try it. If you look at this list and feel that adding one more item to your to-do list would be too much, DON'T DO IT! There might come a time when one of these practices will be something you can do.

If there's any one of these hacks I would say is the *most* important, it's sleep. With the women I coach, sleep is the thing which usually causes the most issues, especially with weight, energy, and mental wellness. If you aren't getting adequate sleep, *everything* will suffer, including your metabolism.

Get sleep in order first, and so many other things will follow.

I would start with a magnesium supplement. My second recommendation would be blue-blocking glasses, since so many people have issues with this and don't even realize it. Once you're steadily getting around eight hours of sleep per night, you'll start to feel like a new person, and the stalls will break and your energy will skyrocket. I would also suggest that for those who have chronic issues with falling asleep, try eating a white plate in the evening before bed; carbs naturally slow us down a bit, so use them to help slow down and relax and then get ready for a good night's sleep.

BAD BIOHACKS I *DON'T* RECOMMEND:

- *Fat bombs:* unnecessary. For those who might be unfamiliar with the term, a fat bomb is just a small snack of highly concentrated fat, used by people following a ketogenic eating plan to help get into ketosis or keep their bodies in ketosis. From my perspective, though, if you're trying to put your body into ketosis, you want your body to burn your *own* fat, not additional fat you're ingesting.

- *Butter overload just because*: again with the butter! It's fine to put butter on things, but please, for the love of God, DO NOT just eat a stick of butter. WHY? I actually saw this on Instagram with the hashtag "#healthy."

Yes, butter is great, but you don't need to eat a whole stick of it. Try to think about Grandma when you do this. Would Grandma eat a stick of butter? Put your butter on some veggies and get the full health benefit. Bonus points if you add some garlic or another detoxifier, like onions.

- *Chasing ketones*: I think a lot of people are confused about ketones. First, your body will go naturally into ketosis if you're doing any sort of window fasting around the 16-18 hour mark. Second, our ancestors regularly experienced this—it's only in our modern era that this stopped happening. You don't need to take extra ketones and, in fact, I just read that Dr. Benjamin Bikman out of BYU thinks taking those extra ketones causes fat to stay put rather than help it burn off. So although external ketones might provide additional energy, they might also hurt us in the long run. If you're testing your blood for ketones, it's also important to note that higher ketones don't necessarily mean you're burning more fat, or are in a deeper state of ketosis. Please stop worrying about this and just focus on how you feel! That is absolutely the best indicator of your health and how your body is functioning. I'm always surprised when I ask someone how they're feeling and they tell me they don't know. Get in touch with your body so you know exactly how you feel, rather than worry about numbers.

- *Dry fasting*: For those of you unfamiliar with the term "dry fasting," it's when you don't have any contact with water at all while in a fast. That means you don't bathe or shower, you don't wash your hands or brush your teeth, and you don't drink any water at all. I've seen a few places on the Internet where people are talking about doing this for three days, and that's extreme to the point that it can actually kill you. Yes, *kill* you. Now, here's the really crazy part about this—I've heard people in the health community refer to this practice in a very nonchalant way, so let me restate my point: extended dry fasting can *KILL* you. For those who might already be a little dehydrated, this will kill you even faster. Please don't do this. Water fasting is safe and effective, and has no adverse side effects…like DEATH!

JASINDA'S SPECIAL "NON-BIO" HACKS

I have a few special life hacks I use; I know I've mentioned some of these before, but I think they bear repeating.

- DINNER HACK: Candles and music. I want you to get on Amazon right now and get some cheap metal candlesticks and a big box of utility candles. Put them on your table as soon as they come and light them every single night when you have dinner. I also want you to play some nice soothing jazz or piano music. We also like to play music from the country of origin of whatever we're eating that night. My kids love it and look forward to it each and every night. We also go around the table and each person tells their joy or blessing of the day. It might seem awkward when you first start, but this will become a highlight of your day.

- PADDED BRAS and BIKINIS: Okay, so if you read the last book, you know I had my breasts reduced and lifted. Well, since then I've lost more weight and now I have nothing there. My fourteen-year-old son has more on his chest than I do, but I'm totally okay with it. Since I've only recently been without boobs I'm just now learning about them: one word, BOMBSHELL! I just wear a nice padded bra from Victoria's Secret, and so many people comment on how nice my boobs look. I don't wear them all the time, but there are outfits that just fit better when I have the boobs to match the booty, if you know what I mean. The other bonus is that I'm pretty sure those bras could save my life as a flotation device. #bonus

- BUBBLES ARE YOUR BEST FRIEND: I'm sure many of you have been told that when you think you're hungry you're actually just thirsty. I really believe this, as I've experienced it in my fasting. Most people are in a state of dehydration all of the time. When you fast you'll really need to stay on top of it. Toxins are being released from your body as you fast—they're literally releasing from your fat as you are fasting and the best way to flush them out is with water. You don't want all of those toxins just sitting in there, do you? You know what a huge fan I am of LaCroix, and with fasting we need to stick to the plain, unflavored version. When I do experience that feeling of hunger when ghrelin (the hormone that tells your body you're hungry) is peaking, I just grab a can of Pure LaCroix and the bubbles mimic that full feeling in my tummy. I know people say drinking plain water is tough, but experiment with a few different types of water to find one that works for you. You may need a fancy glass with some ice and a straw, or a brand of water that comes in a glass bottle versus a can, or maybe you need to leave your can out for a bit so it isn't so bubbly. Don't give up trying until you've found something that really works for you!

- PLANT A GARDEN: I know not everyone can easily do this but I really want to encourage you to try, even if you can only do a small herb garden on your balcony. Gardens are magical, and eating food you grow yourself is unicorn-level magical. Your garden doesn't have to be complicated, either. Just pick two or three of your favorite herbs or veggies and start there. If your family loves cucumber, lettuce, and basil, you can easily put them into a nice little container garden right on your back porch. I remember when I was a kid almost all of our neighbors had gardens. In fact, on a late summer afternoon, everyone would go into their backyards and check on their garden, water, and chat. The men would congregate to chat, drink a beer, and trade vegetables with each other—this was back in the day when you knew your neighbors. I think there's something therapeutic about getting your hands dirty and watching something you planted grow and then eating it. Heck, I'll even go a step further and encourage you to think about a community garden. Maybe you have a neighbor or friend who might want to do this with you. You may not be able to take on the time and responsibility of doing it all yourself, but if you have a friend to do it with, it could be something you could manage together. Our church has an awesome community garden. Maybe you can share what you grow! I can't tell you how much work and fun our family has experienced in our garden. Just ask my mom about the giant wasp nest she found hiding behind the tomatoes! Okay, don't ask her that, but there are memories to be made here, too, my friends. Just start small, especially if you tend to kill anything green. Enlist your kids to help. You can do it!

A few quick words of final encouragement before I move into the FAQs and recipes and such; this is a process, so take it slow. Remember our mantras: One day at a time, one meal at a time; give yourself and your body grace; you can do it! Fasting is a muscle, which requires exercise to strengthen, so don't get discouraged if it's a little challenging at first.

Fasting isn't just a physical game—it's mental, too, so get your head in the process. Be aware of what your body is telling you, and listen to it. Remember that tomorrow is always another day, and another day to restart your fast if you need to break for any reason.

As I laid out in earlier chapters, fasting also can be about more than just not eating. It can help you simplify your life. It can teach you how to strip away distractions and needless clutter, how to focus your attention on the things that DO matter—your health, and your family.

You can do it! I've made that the title of these books, and I've repeated it throughout—you *can* do it! You're worth it, and your health is worth it!

Frequently Asked Questions

(AND ANSWERS)

BELOW ARE SOME OF THE MOST FREQUENTLY ASKED questions that come my way. As I've coached women, I've found that we all tend to deal with many of the same things and often have the same questions. I'm posting these FAQs here in the hope that the questions might help you. Please remember that I'm not a doctor and anything answered here is simply based on my personal experience, and that I always recommend talking with your doctor about your health before you try anything new.

Q: I'm scared to fast; how should I start?
A: Fasting is a "muscle," so to speak, and it takes time and practice to get it working. I recommend starting small and

just try to eliminate breakfast for a while to see how you do and how you feel. With most things we attempt in terms of diet and exercise, we do too much at the start and overwhelm ourselves, and then end up feeling like we've failed because we took on too much too soon. Please, do NOT just jump head-first into the waters of fasting by trying a 3-day fast your very first time. Just take it one step at a time, keep a journal, and you'll find your rhythm.

Q: Do you think I should wait until I'm close to my goal weight before I begin fasting?

A: This is a tricky one for me, because I was pretty close to my original goal weight when I started fasting. I've seen people really do well with it at every stage of their journey, so I would say that as long as you aren't pregnant, breastfeeding, or underweight, you should be fine to try some fasting at whatever weight you are. I do think that waiting until I got into my health groove with my eating habits did help make fasting a bit easier. When you don't have to worry about craving or detoxifying from sugars and refined carbohydrates, fasting is much easier. One step at a time, as always, but also remember that one size doesn't fit all when it comes to health. If you try window fasting and you feel horrible and hangry, give it some time and try again later.

Q: If I'm trying to fast for autophagy can I have coffee?

A: No. If you want the full benefit of autophagy, you need to stick to water and salt *only*. I know this is hard, but it's necessary and worth it. If you're not feeling good, stop and try again later—that's always the rule with fasting, no matter what. Dr. Fung thinks that autophagy really kicks in between eighteen to thirty-six hours into a fast, so that's a good goal line.

Q: Can I work out in a fasted state?

A: Yes! Jack and I do this all the time. When you work out while fasting, you're burning fat versus glycogen. I have the most focus and the best energy for working out when I'm fasted. I've actually done a 5K run after fasting for several days and I felt fantastic. I also think strength training sessions are great done while fasting. We've seen some great definition in our muscles since doing our fasted workouts. Jack probably wouldn't attempt a marathon-length run without some help from carbohydrates, but pretty much everything else works well while fasting.

Q: Is it okay for my kids to fast?

A: No, I wouldn't recommend fasting for children. Since they're still growing it's important they eat regularly. It's also important that they are eating the right things—a steady diet of processed food is not doing them any favors. This doesn't mean I force my kids to eat if they aren't hungry, but we always tell them they need to eat so they can get big and strong like Mommy and Daddy.

Q: Can I take my vitamins when I'm fasting?

A: I don't. I think it's best to take your vitamins and supplements with or between meals. There is also some evidence that the coating on vitamins could actually stop your fast, so best to be safe and wait until you're done with your fast before resuming your vitamin regimen.

Q: What supplements do you take?

A: I take a few things on a regular basis. I still take a multivitamin and a probiotic every day, but I try to get as many of my nutrients from food. Because I have nutritional issues, I try to stay on top of that because I start feeling bad pretty fast if my iron, electrolytes, or minerals are out of whack. I also take a wellness supplement that helps with my adrenals. I started taking 5-HTP during a very stressful time, and I found it was great for me as it helps the body produce serotonin. If you have anxiety, panic attacks, sleep issues, or minor depression, you should talk with your doctor and get his or her advice. I hope I won't always need these things, but I also know that sometimes, since my health has been in pretty bad shape for so long, giving myself grace by taking a supplement to help is totally okay.

Q: Will fasting slow my metabolism?

A: Fasting has been shown to *increase* metabolism. Once you hit three days of fasting you reach a peak where your metabolism increases and autophagy peaks as well. This is another reason why I think I a 3-day fast is optimal to see great benefits.

Q: Are you still running?

A: Yes, but not as much as I was. I'll be running a 5k with my mother, sister, and daughter that we're all really excited about, and I'm doing a half marathon in May. I've taken to doing bodyweight exercises—I love planks, lunges, push-ups, squats, jumps, and crunches. I also really love stretching and yoga and walks and dancing. I try to find ways to exercise daily and it's often with my kids or Jack, we might just take a walk together, or dance around the kitchen. I would say we do a family run every month or two, and I do cardio maybe once a week. I do yoga at least once a week, and Jack and I do bodyweight exercises for maybe fifteen to twenty minutes two or three times a week. I firmly believe exercise really only accounts for maybe 10 percent of your health and body composition, so I focus on my eating and nutrition, and think of my movement as icing on the health cake.

Q: What is the biggest mistake you've seen people making with the #wilderway lifestyle?

A: The biggest mistake I see is people eating too many approved packaged foods, like Dreamfields pasta, Mission wraps, Halo Top, Lily's, Dr. John's, and Quest bars. These are all approved and okay with my plan, but they *are* packaged, and they do have some ingredients I reserve for only occasional use. I've found many of the ladies who get stuck or stalled for long periods of time are indulging in these things daily, and that can really become an issue pretty quickly. I try to reserve any packaged foods for special treats and they are not something I eat every day. The best things for you, nutritionally, don't come in a package, they come from the earth. Try to stick to those things on a daily basis and you will see continued results.

Q: Where can I get more info about that Enneagram thing you were talking about?
A: www.enneagraminstitute.com

Q: What is ketosis, and what are ketones?
A: Ketosis is a metabolic process where the body, lacking glucose—which is the human body's go-to source of fuel and energy—begins burning body fat for fuel instead; ketones are simply an organic molecular compound produced naturally when the body is in a state of ketosis.

Q: Will you be doing group fasting challenges?
A: Fasting is personal, and it should be intuitive, so I won't do an actual "group challenge," but I may do individual fasting challenges in a group setting. Sometimes fasting goes exactly as planned, and other times it's just not the right day, space, or time for you to be fasting. Women are such complex creatures, and as I've progressed with my health journey I've discovered how much my body is ruled by hormones. I have one week in my cycle where fasting is almost effortless, while other days I know I need to stop because my body just isn't having it. I know I've said this a million times already, but it's *SO* important for us to listen to our bodies and be tuned into them so we know when it's a time meant for feasting and

when it's a time meant for fasting. Fasting is a personal, solitary practice. Fast, Journal, Pray, Meditate.

> If you haven't downloaded the CLUE app already, do it right now! It REALLY helps tune you into your cycle. There are days when you wake up and your body is ready to fast and other days the struggle is too real. Don't fight your body. Listen, and do whatever is best for you. It would be impossible for me to set a challenge where people might feel pressured or pushed not to listen to themselves.

Q: Why does my weight keep going up and down while I'm fasting?

A: This is the money question—I get it more frequently than any other. Your weight is going to fluctuate. My weight has a range of about ten pounds depending on what I'm eating (white plates cause water retention), where I am in my cycle, and whether I've been fasting or not. My weight usually goes up about five pounds for a few days during ovulation, *and* during my period. This might sound like a lot to people, but I don't worry about it at all. Some women worry about gaining two pounds. TWO POUNDS! Guys, two pounds could vanish from one good poop! Let me just say that, for most of us, our weight fluctuates due to our natural, normal biology. Please, stop freaking out about this. Get some rest, move, make good choices, listen to your body, and keep at it. All will be well, I promise.

Q: Do you ever cheat with food?

A: Man, the cheat question is a hot topic. I personally don't cheat because I can't even think about how bad I would feel if I did. If I have something with the *slightest* amount of sugar in it, I just feel like total crap, so I refuse to do that to myself anymore. There's really nothing I can't figure out a way to modify or adjust so I can enjoy it. I was even able to modify my grandmother's favorite vanilla wafer cake this year and I had a pretty big piece! If you feel like you really *must* have something, such as a few bites of cake at your niece's wedding or whatever, I would suggest you just start fresh the next day with a really fatty black plate, since that will help bring your blood sugar down and cut out some of the carb cravings you might have. I don't believe in guilt or shame with food choices. Just focus on the next meal and make the best choices you can.

Q: How do you deal with social situations when food is being served?

A: I always carry a big purse, and it always has things in it I can eat. If I'm going to a wedding or party, there's usually some protein I can focus on. I might remove the breading from the chicken, or just do a giant salad with a big side of veggies and then, if I'm still hungry, I'll eat a protein bar, nuts, dark chocolate, or meat sticks from my purse. Girl, I have *no* shame and I will totally pull out a meat stick from my purse. At my 20th high school reunion I pulled out some keto cookies and passed them around for friends to try. I've even had people emailing me to say that they carry Mission wraps in their purse when they travel. I love it and I think it's great to be prepared. I wasn't a Girl Scout, but there's something to learn from them. Maybe we can figure out some #wilderway girl patches!

Q: Won't any diet that's low glycemic and reduces insulin work as a weight-loss program?

A: Yep! This is why I see people being successful on Keto, or paleo, Whole 30, or things like stevia-sweetened shakes, or even Weight Watchers. I think the biggest difference is between "going on a diet" and "changing your *lifestyle*." These things are all going to work as long as they're sustainable.

For most people the big lure is how quickly they can lose the most amount of weight. But from the data I've seen, and what I've experienced myself, unless something can be maintained for life there's going to be a point when anything can fail. It's important to be able to find not just a diet that will work to take off weight, but to find something you do not just for a season, but also for life. This often means working hard to replace things we know are our downfall. Maybe it's the donuts we eat when we are stressed, or the tub of Ben and Jerry ice cream we have when the in-laws are on the way. Whatever it is, we have to plan for those things, because they'll still exist even after we have reached our "happy weight." Life isn't suddenly going to be perfect the moment we reach some magical number on the scale. We have to find ways to cope with stress, and create safety nets, so when we experience those stressful times we maintain our lifestyle and cope in ways that don't become unhealthy and self-abusive. I think the information I've shared with you in these three books should allow you to figure out a way to reach and maintain a healthy lifestyle. But, if not, I encourage you to keep working on it, keep reading, keep advocating for yourself with your doctors, and keep trying to find what works best for you!

Q: Do you tell people when you are fasting?
A: NOPE! I think there's still a stigma with fasting. I know most people don't really get it, and if you tell someone who once had a cousin who was anorexic they're going to give you fifty reasons why they think you're becoming anorexic. I'm a pretty private person anyway, but with things like this I think it's always better to keep it to myself unless there is a reason to let someone know. My kids often ask me about it and, of course, I always tell them if I'm fasting and for how long and why. But with extended family or acquaintances, I wouldn't recommend discussing it unless you're prepared to hear a lot of opinions, some of which might not be very favorable. At parties I always have a drink in my hand. I've gone to several events where people have been eating—church events, fundraisers, a school function, year-end beach parties, a concert with friends—while I was fasting and not a single person noticed or said a thing. I do want to point out that if, for any reason, at any of these events, I decide I want to enjoy some food, I absolutely break my fast and eat. I also don't think it's a great idea to plan a fast at a big event like a wedding, a retirement party, a birthday

party, or some other type of big family celebration. Later on you might regret not eating with everyone and I think it's important to enjoy those moments. You can always fast another day. Enjoy those times and fast when it works best for your life and your family.

Q: Do you get constipated when you fast?
A: I do see my regularity go from every day to maybe every other day but, if anything, my poop is softer and easier to pass. Even with my extended fasts I continued to go the bathroom pretty regularly. It's really important to have those veggies with lots of fiber during your feasting times to keep your bowels in good health. I eat leafy greens at almost every meal, and I haven't needed to add any additional fiber. In fact, my chronic hemorrhoids that occurred as a result of a previous birthing experience (not saying any names... ahem—child #5!) have improved since I started fasting a year ago. Proof that inflammation has continued to improve in all corners of my body. Sorry—TMI!

Q: How many white plates should I have per week?
A: That is totally personal. I think you need to experiment and know what's best for you. At the place I am at today, I like to save up my carbs for the weekend. Black plates and fasting really help me during the weekdays, and then I usually do kefir, oatmeal, some sprouted bread, or cereal on the weekend. I occasionally have sweet potatoes too, although we seem to eat more of those in the fall and summer months. I am a tiny

bit addicted to kefir, so if I am going to pick one carb to have it would be kefir and I might even have it a few times on a weekend. I love it that much! I also love a good sprouted bread peanut butter and jelly sandwich as my big splurge grey plate meal—those are my all time favorite! During my period I probably eat more white plates too; it really just depends on how I'm feeling. That is one of my favorite things about this lifestyle—I mix it up and do what works best for me. Keep experimenting! There's no wrong answer.

Q: When will I stop being cranky when I fast?

A: Well, this is something that we really worried about with Jack. Mr. Crankypants was *super* cranky when he first tried fasting. I mean, super cranky! I think it just takes some time for your body to adjust. I also think if you're already following a low carb, low sugar diet your body will deal with fasting better, because you won't have the unstable blood sugar swings to contend with. I also think making sure you have a really fatty, heavy black plate meal before starting your fast really helps, too. So make sure to pick your favorite fat-rich black plate before you start. I usually have a few fried eggs in butter with an avocado.

Q: Is there anything else I can add to my fasting beverages that won't actually break the fast?

A: Yes; I will sometimes add a lemon or lime to my Pure LaCroix when I'm fasting, and it's just about the best thing ever. I will also add some ACV (Apple Cider Vinegar) once a day, too. Some people will add a tiny bit of MCT oil to coffee to tide them over during an extended fast. I really try to fast as clean as possible, so the day before I start I prefer to have some heavy whipping cream and MCT oil in my coffee, but then once I'm actually into my fast I just take my coffee or tea black. You could also add a bit of cinnamon to your coffee or tea for flavor if that appeals to you.

Q: How do you talk with your kids about fasting and about their health and body image? I'm worried I'm not saying or doing the things I should.

A: I think I could probably devote an entire chapter to this one question, so if this runs long just bear with me. I think the best way I can answer this is to tell you what I think you *shouldn't* do. I *don't* think you should ever speak negatively about health or body TO your kids, or AROUND your kids. There isn't a time in my childhood when I didn't feel shame and negativity about my body—not from my parents so much as from doctors and society in general. I got horrible looks and comments from adults even when I was five or six years old. My advice is to always talk positively to your kids about how amazing their bodies are, and how important it is to take care of our bodies by what we put into it. Talk to them about how we can make good choices and not so great choices, and that it's okay if we sometimes make bad choices, but we should try to make more good than bad. We can praise them when we see them making those good choices, but I don't think we should scold, punish, or shame them if they aren't making the best ones. Every Sunday our church has sugary treats for the kids, and every Sunday my kids make the choice not to have them, so we always take them to brunch where they get unlimited bacon, sausage, eggs, and berries. They love it! Did I mention kids eat free at this brunch, and every adult brunch comes with complimentary champagne? #winning! Truly, though, I think we should be honest with our kids about health. Jack and I are always in constant conversation with our kids about health. We talk openly about our own struggles and why we're doing what we're doing. When I started fasting, my kids had so many questions. Why wasn't I eating? When would I be eating again? Was it okay for them to fast? Why, or why not? Is it ever okay for them to skip a meal? What happens to people who go too long without eating? I swear my seven-year-old had about thirty questions right off the top of his head. I love it when my kids have questions for me, and it worries me when they're too quiet. Sit down and have some positive conversations with your kids that emphasize good health and good choices. I also make sure my kids understand that not everyone has to make the same choices as they do; we don't want them shaming friends for eating a candy bar!

Q: If I eat the same amount of calories during my window that I would've eaten during the day over three meals, how will I lose weight? Isn't it the same thing in the end?

A: No. When you eat during a window, your body has all that other time you aren't eating to rest in a state of low insulin, so the body can engage in the process of burning up all of your fat for fuel. Think of it as extended fat burning versus little spurts of time when fat isn't able to burn off because your insulin is too high. We get *so* much more bang from our fat burning bucks when we eat during a limited window. It's fat burning magic when our body is running at high efficiency while fasting!

Q: What shouldn't I have during a fast? Can I chew gum or have a mint?

A: You want to stick to water, salt, black coffee, and clear tea. I brush my teeth, but I don't recommend any gum, mints, sweeteners, flavoring—even flavored LaCroix—cream, or oil. The cleaner you fast the better the results you'll see.

Q: Do you still think protein should be the main focus of all plates?

A: Yes, protein is always my focus. I try to stick to around a gram of protein for every pound of my ideal weight—so if my happy weight is 180 lbs, I'll eat around 180 grams of protein per day. I use fats and carbs as a sort of leverage with my metabolism and hormones. At this point in my journey, I know when I need carbohydrates, and I know when fats are best. I hope if you've read all three of my books you're getting a better understanding with that too. It does take time and effort to figure out exactly what combinations fuel your body best, but once you do, your body will thank you. Take the time and do it right!

More of Jasinda's Favorite Things

- La Croix—Dude, have you tried the Key Lime flavor?

- Zevia—Root beer is life!

- Keto Cookies—Peanut butter is my favorite

- Zella pants from Nordstrom—I wear these from yoga to the street

- The Clue app—This baby will track your period so you know exactly when it's coming

- Calia by Carrie—I really love her motivational tank tops

- Victoria's Secret—Very SEXY and Bombshell bras

- The Mercari app—For clothes to buy and sell as you change sizes

- Evereve Trendsend clothing box—This has really saved me from myself time and time again. They send you several outfits in your size (even better if you send them your measurements), at your budget (yes, you can tell them just clearance items), and you just keep what you like and send the rest back. I've yet to have them send me something that I don't absolutely love.

- Kettle & Fire Bone Broth—Because who has time to make their own bone broth? This one is great!

- Alaffia and Acure—Natural and organic bath and body products.

- Hush and Dotti—Organic makeup. I LOVE their cheek and lip color, lip gloss and eyeliner. LOVE!

- Epsom salt—I love the EPSOAK 3-pack bundle on Amazon. Taking a nice, warm bath with salt during a fast is awesome. Dr. Teals is also great.

- SPANX!—I don't know how you can lose over one hundred pounds and not love SPANX. They hold everything in so nicely. If you haven't tried the new arm tights, grab a pair!

- Grounds and Hounds coffee—I love this coffee, and every purchase supports a great cause.

- DRY FARMS WINE—The best wine ever. We have tested this against all other wines and not only do we stay in ketosis, but we have no issues with blood sugar. It rocks!

Additional Resources and Reading

APPS:

- FASTING SECRET (countdown or hourly fasting tracker)

- SOBER TIME (fasting clock)

- WINDOW FASTING (window fasting tracker)

- CLUE (cycle tracking)

- Calm (meditation)

- 10% Happier (meditation)

- Waterminder (water intake reminder)

- Yoga Studio

BOOKS:

- *The Complete Guide to Fasting* by Dr. Jason Fung

- *The Metabolic Approach to Cancer* by Dr. Nasha Winters, ND, L. Ac, FABNO, and Jess Higgins Kelley, MNT

- *Keto* by Maria Emmerich and Craig Emmerich. All of Maria's cookbooks are great for black plates. Our family really loves her restaurant favorites cookbook.

- *The Road Back To You: An Enneagram Journey To Self-Discovery* by Ian Cron and Susanne Stabile

- *Clutterfree With Kids* by Joshua Becker

- *21 Days of Eating Mindfully* by Lorrie Jones MBSR BSN CYI. I really loved this book and I believe working on being mindful in all things is an excellent practice.

- *Bacon & Butter: The Ultimate Ketogenic Diet Cookbook* by Celby Richoux (black plates)

- *The Keto Diet* by Leanne Vogel

- *Keto Essentials* by Vanessa Spina

- *Keto Comfort Foods* by Maria Emmerich

BLOGS, PODCASTS, AND VIDEOS:

- *The Obesity Code with Dr. Jason Fung, and Megan Ramos of Intensive Dietary Management.* **Special thanks to Megan for answering my questions and talking with me about her experiences with fasting and the IDM program. You rock!**

- *High Intensity Health Radio with Mike Mutzel, MSc*

- *The Minimalists Podcast, with Joshua Fields Millburn and Ryan Nicodemus*

- *10% Happier With Dan Harris*

- Yoga by Candace

- Yoga With Adriene

Recipes

IN OUR ONGOING QUEST TO FIND DELICIOUS, EASY, AND nutritious meals and treats, we created these recipes, almost all of which are black plates. When I'm at a loss for something to make, I go to my giant cookbook collection or Pinterest for inspiration. We eat mostly black plates during the week, which limits things a little, making it that much easier—we just go back to the tried and true family favorites time and again. We hope these recipes inspire you to go back to your family favorites and find ways you might be able to make them healthier for your family! Enjoy!

BABY REE'S YUMMY GUMMIES
(INSPIRED BY THE KETO DIET BY LEANNE VOGEL)

Ingredients
- 1 ¼ cups boiling water, divided
- 3 tea bags
- ¼ cup gelatin
- ¼ cup lemon juice
- a splash of flavored extract (your choice)
- powdered or liquid sweetener (to taste)
- 1 scoop collagen

Directions: Steep tea bags in ¾ cups boiling water. Remove the bags and whisk in gelatin, sweetener, and extract. Then whisk in the remaining ½ cup boiling water and the lemon juice. If more sweetener is needed, add that now. Pour into silicone molds and refrigerate about an hour to set. Remove from molds and store in an airtight container in the fridge. These are her favorite thing in the whole world! Find some fun molds and get the kids involved in making them.

- We like strawberry tea with strawberry extract, raspberry tea with raspberry extract, and lemon tea with lemon extract. But feel free to get creative.
- If you aren't a tea person, you can use flavored extract instead. You just need to keep adding more until it's to your desired taste. And to make it more fun for the kids, we like to add a couple drops of natural food coloring to make them specific colors to match the flavors. We love orange and lime this way.

EGG CUPS

Makes 12 egg cups

Ingredients
- 9 eggs
- 1 cup cheddar cheese
- 1 tsp seasoning of choice (we use Flavorgod everything)
- Spinach
- Bacon crumbles or sliced sausages

Directions: Preheat your oven to 350 degrees; spray your muffin tins with coconut spray or use liners. Place your sausages or bacon in the bottom of your muffin tin and sprinkle in some spinach. Now put your eggs, cheese, and seasoning in the blender. Mix on high until well blended. Pour mixture into your prepared muffin tins. Bake for 20-25 minutes. These can be eaten immediately or stored for later. If storing for later: Once cooled, store in an airtight container in the fridge. Take out however many you want and microwave. Enjoy!

CHERRY SHAKE*

Serves 1-2

Ingredients
- ½ cup cottage cheese
- 1 1/3 cups cashew milk
- ¼ cup heavy cream
- 1 ½ tsp cherry extract
- 1 tsp almond extract
- 4-5 strawberries (for color)
- 1 TBSP sweetener of choice
- 1 scoop collagen
- 1 scoop vanilla protein powder
- 1 cup ice
- Cocoa nibs for crunchiness (optional)

Directions: Put all ingredients except ice and cocoa nibs in blender. Blend on high to make nice and fluffy. Add ice and cocoa nibs and blend until smooth. Pour and enjoy!

BETTER THAN CANDY SHAKE*

Makes one shake

Ingredients
- 1 cup cashew milk
- ¼ cup heavy cream
- 1 scoop chocolate protein powder
- 3 TBSP powdered peanut butter
- 2 TBSP cocoa powder
- ¼ tsp caramel extract
- ¼ tsp butter extract
- ¼ tsp glucomannan
- 2 TBSP sweetener of choice
- 1 scoop collagen
- 1 cup ice

Directions: Place everything except ice in a blender. Blend on high until well mixed. Add ice and blend until smooth. Pour into your glass and enjoy.

JASINDA'S FAVORITE RASPBERRY SHAKE*

Makes one shake

Ingredients
- 1 cup cashew milk
- ½ cup heavy cream
- ½ scoop vanilla protein powder
- ½ cup raspberries (fresh or frozen)
- 5 drops liquid stevia

Directions: Blend it all together in your blender. Add ice if desired. Pour into your favorite glass and enjoy!

*You can use whichever berry you choose. My littlest princess loves blueberry, and my little boys love strawberry.

PEANUT BUTTER SHAKE*

Makes one shake

Ingredients
- 1 cup cashew milk
- ½ cup heavy cream
- ½ scoop vanilla protein
- 3 TBSP powdered Peanut butter
- ½ tsp vanilla extract
- 5 drops liquid stevia
- 1 cup ice
- We sometimes throw a handful of our favorite berries in this to make it a PB&J shake. YUMM!!

Directions: Blend all ingredients except ice together until fluffy. Add ice and blend until smooth. Pour and enjoy!

*With all of these shakes, you can use additional cashew or almond milk in place of the heavy cream.

KING TOM'S TURKEY PIZZA

Makes 1 pizza

Ingredients
- 1 pound ground turkey
- ½ cup parmesan cheese
- 1 tsp Italian seasoning
- Pizza sauce
- Cheese
- Additional toppings of choice

Directions: Preheat oven to 350 degrees. In a large bowl, mix seasoning, parmesan, and turkey using your hands. Roll meat mixture out on greased pizza stone. Bake for 20-25 minutes, or until cooked through. Once the meat is cooked, remove from oven, spread your sauce on it, and top with cheese and your choice of toppings. Toss back in the oven for about 10 minutes until the cheese is melted.

Get creative! This is a family favorite.

PERFECT PANCAKES

Serves 3

Ingredients
- 1 cup almond flour
- 1 TBSP sweetener
- ¼ tsp salt
- 1 tsp baking powder
- 2 eggs
- 1/8 cup heavy cream
- 1/8 cup sparkling water
- ½ tsp vanilla extract
- 2 TBSP coconut oil, melted

Directions: Preheat griddle on medium heat. In a large bowl, mix almond flour, sweetener, salt, and baking powder. Make a well in the center of your dry ingredients and add eggs, heavy cream, sparkling water, vanilla, and oil. Spray griddle with cooking spray before cooking. Use ¼ to 1/3 cup batter per pancake.

Variations:
- Chocolate - Add a couple tablespoons of cocoa powder.
- Peanut butter - Add some powdered peanut butter.
- Cinnamon – Add a touch of cinnamon

Again guys, get creative. Have fun in the kitchen!

WILDER KIDS BERRY "YOGURT" BITES

Ingredients
- 4 TBSP Butter
- 4 TBSP coconut oil
- 2 oz cream cheese
- 4 TBSP heavy cream
- ¼ cup your favorite berries (chopped)
- 1 tsp vanilla extract
- A couple drops of liquid stevia (to taste)

Directions: In a microwaveable bowl, melt butter, cream cheese, and oil. Now mix in the heavy cream. Pour into a blender or use a hand mixer and add the vanilla, stevia, and berries. Blend until smooth. Pour into ice cube trays or silicone molds and place in the freezer. You can freeze them overnight or just for a couple of hours. Remove from the molds or ice cube trays and store in an airtight container in the freezer.

WILDER KIDS LEMON "YOGURT" BITES

Ingredients
- 4 TBSP butter
- 4 TBSP coconut oil
- 2 oz cream cheese
- 4 TBSP heavy cream
- 2 TBSP lemon juice
- 1 tsp lemon extract
- Liquid stevia (to taste)

Directions: In a microwave-safe bowl, melt butter, cream cheese, and oil. Stir well. Add heavy cream and mix well. Add lemon juice, lemon extract, and stevia. Mix until smooth, pour into ice cube trays or silicone molds. Set in freezer for two or more hours. Remove from molds and store in an airtight container in the freezer.

CHICKEN TENDERS

Ingredients
- 1 pound chicken tenderloins (or breasts cut into strips)
- ½ cup plain protein powder
- 1 cup parmesan cheese
- 2 tsp seasoning of choice: I usually use garlic, but I also sometimes use Italian, cayenne, salt and pepper, Flavor God everything seasoning, or ranch.
- 2 eggs
- 2 TBSP butter, melted
- Avocado or olive oil for frying

Directions: Pour enough oil in your skillet to cover the bottom of the pan. Heat on medium. In a shallow dish, whisk eggs and melted butter. In another shallow dish combine protein powder, parmesan cheese, and seasoning. Flip your chicken around in the egg wash then do the same in the "breading" to coat it well. Place your chicken tenders in the hot oil. Cook a couple minutes on each side until the internal temperature is 165 degrees. Serve and enjoy!

MOM'S FANCY BREAKFAST MUFFINS

Serves 12

Ingredients
- 1 ½ cups almond flour
- ½ cup flax meal
- ½ cup powdered sweetener
- 2 tsp baking powder
- 1 TBSP cinnamon
- 1 tsp ground cloves
- ½ tsp salt
- 6 eggs
- ½ cup melted coconut oil
- ½ cup heavy cream
- 1 tsp vanilla

Directions: Preheat oven to 350 degrees. In a large bowl, whisk together almond flour, flax meal, sweetener, baking powder, cinnamon, cloves, and salt. Then mix in remaining ingredients. Now, fill your muffin tins about 2/3 full. Bake for about 25 minutes. We tend to prep and cook these, and store them in the fridge for a quick and easy breakfast. When I want to get really fancy I'll frost these with cream cheese and berries. #yum

These are good with cream cheese, butter, almond butter, or peanut butter on top.

Perfect for breakfast on the go, or snacks anytime!

PERFECT PROTEIN BARS
(INSPIRED BY KETO ESSENTIALS BY VANESSA SPINA)

Ingredients
- ½ cup hemp hearts
- ¼ cup sunflower seeds
- ¼ cup pumpkin seeds
- ½ cup almonds chopped
- ½ cup walnuts/pecans chopped
- ¼ cup chia seeds
- ¼ tsp cinnamon
- ¾ cup butter
- 3 TBSP sweetener
- 1 tsp vanilla extract
- ½ tsp liquid stevia
- ¼ tsp salt
- 2 eggs
- 2 TBSP almond butter

Directions: Preheat oven to 350 degrees. Line a 13x9 inch pan, or one of similar size, with parchment paper. In a bowl combine all your seeds and nuts. In a large saucepan, melt cinnamon, butter, and sweeteners. Once completely melted, pour in nuts-and-seeds mixture. Mix in almond butter, eggs, and salt. Pour mixture into parchment paper-lined pan; spread it out to cover the whole pan. Sprinkle some chocolate chips on top and place in the oven for 20 minutes or until golden brown. Let cool completely, cut, and store in the fridge in an airtight container. These are a great snack to take on the go.

BROWNIES

Ingredients

- 1 ½ cups almond flour
- 1 cup sweetener
- 6 TBSP cocoa powder
- 1 tsp baking powder
- ½ tsp salt
- ½ cup butter, melted
- 6 eggs
- 2 tsp vanilla
- ½ cup chocolate chips

Directions: Preheat oven to 350 degrees. In a large bowl, whisk together flour, sweetener, cocoa powder, baking powder, and salt. Add butter, eggs, and vanilla. Whisk until well combined and smooth. Stir in chocolate chips. Pour into a greased 13x9 inch pan. Cook for 30 minutes. Let cool and enjoy every last bite!

WAFFLES

Ingredients
- 5 ½ cups Kodiak Power Cakes mix
- 5 ½ cups water
- 4 eggs
- 2 tsp vanilla

Directions: Preheat your waffle iron. Mix all ingredients in a large bowl until smooth; I like to use a hand mixer. Spray waffle iron with coconut spray, pour batter into waffle iron, and cook until done. This usually makes 9 Belgian waffles. Top with syrup, berries, and whipped cream.

CHEESIEST CHEESEBURGERS SENT STRAIGHT FROM HEAVEN (INSPIRED BY KETO COMFORT FOODSBY MARIA EMMERICH)

Ingredients
- 3 ½ cups shredded sharp cheddar cheese
- 4 TBSP butter
- 2 eggs
- ¼ tsp salt
- 2 pounds ground turkey
- 8 slices of your favorite cheese
- ½ cup pizza sauce
- Pepper and garlic salt to taste

Directions: Preheat oven to 425 degrees. Divide ground turkey into 8 patties. Season patties with garlic salt and pepper. Cook in a skillet on medium heat until cooked through. While the burgers are cooking, in a large microwave-safe bowl, combine butter and shredded cheese. Melt on high in one-minute increments until cheese is melted. Add the almond flour, salt, and egg. Using your hands, knead it like dough. Split dough into 8 balls. Roll each ball out between two pieces of parchment paper. Once rolled out, place a burger in the center of the dough, top with a tablespoon of pizza sauce and a slice of cheese, fold the sides of the dough up and over to fully enclose the burger patty, and place on a sheet pan or a pizza stone. Once all 8 are ready, place in the oven for 10-15 minutes or until dough is starting to brown. We like to dip these in True Made Foods Vegetable Ketchup; this stuff is amazing! These are another family favorite.

STUFFED MEATBALLS

Makes about 10 large meatballs

Ingredients
- 1 pound ground turkey
- 1 egg
- 2 tsp Italian seasoning
- ¼ cup grated parmesan
- Mozzarella cut into chunks
- 1 cup tomato sauce

Directions: Preheat oven to 400 degrees. In a medium-sized, bowl use your hands to mix all the ingredients except the mozzarella and tomato sauce. Once mixed, roll the meat into balls around a chunk of the mozzarella. Place your meatballs into a greased 9x11 inch baking dish. Pour the tomato sauce over the top. Place in the oven for 25-30 minutes, or until cooked through. Internal temperature should be 165. Protip: we get our mozzarella chunks from Costco

CURRY CHICKEN
(INSPIRED BY BREAD AND WINE BY SHAUNA NIEQUIST)

Ingredients

- ¼ cup almond flour
- 2 TBSP curry powder
- 1 tsp salt
- ¼ tsp cayenne pepper
- 3 pounds boneless chicken breasts
- 4 TBSP olive or avocado oil
- 2 cloves garlic, chopped
- 1 red onion, chopped
- 1 TBSP fresh ginger, chopped
- 1 red bell pepper, chopped
- 4 cups chicken broth
- one green apple
- 2 Roma tomatoes, chopped
- 1 TBSP lime juice
- 3 TBSP fresh cilantro, chopped
- 3 TBSP fresh basil, chopped
-

Directions: Mix together flour, curry powder, salt, and cayenne pepper. Toss chicken into flour mixture and turn to coat well. Pour 2 tablespoons oil into a skillet, add chicken, and cook on medium-high heat until browned, usually about 5 minutes on each side. In another skillet, add the other 2 tablespoons of oil and cook garlic, red onion, ginger, and red pepper until onions are golden, or about 4 minutes. Once the chicken is done, add the cooked vegetables and the chicken broth to the pan of chicken breasts. Simmer until the chicken is cooked and the broth is reduced by 1/4. Add tomatoes and apples. Simmer until heated through. Garnish with lime juice, cilantro, and basil. Serve over brown rice or with a salad.

VANILLA MUG CAKE

Ingredients
- 3 TBSP almond flour
- 2 TBSP sweetener
- 1 egg
- 1/2 TBSP butter, melted
- 1/2 TBSP sour cream
- 1/8 tsp salt
- ¼ tsp vanilla
- ¼ tsp baking powder
- 1 TBSP chocolate chips

Directions: Combine all your ingredients in a mug. Mix well. Microwave on high for 2 minutes. Remove from microwave and top with a spoonful of cream cheese and more chocolate chips. YUM!

BAGELS

Ingredients

- 3 cups almond flour
- 2 TBSP baking powder
- 5 cups grated mozzarella
- 4 oz cream cheese
- 4 eggs, beaten
- Seasoning of choice. We like Everything Seasoning by FlavorGod.

Directions: Preheat oven to 400 degrees. In a large bowl, combine mozzarella and cream cheese. Microwave in one-minute increments until cheeses are melted. Add flour, baking powder, and eggs. Knead the dough with your hands—warning: it will be very sticky. Once the dough is completely mixed, separate into 8 parts. Form a long "log" shape with each part of the dough and then make a bagel shape and place on a baking sheet lined with parchment paper. Sprinkle seasoning of choice on top. Bake for 10-15 minutes, or until golden brown.

Our favorite ways to eat these bagels are:

- Topped with cream cheese or almond butter
- Made into an egg, cheese, and bacon breakfast sandwich
- Cut in half, placed on a baking sheet, and topped with pizza sauce, mozzarella cheese, and pepperoni; place in the oven until cheese is melted.

PLAIN CHEESECAKE WITH VARIATIONS

Makes 1 cheesecake

Ingredients
- (2) 8oz. packages cream cheese, softened
- 2 eggs
- 1 tsp vanilla extract
- ½ cup sweetener
- 1 piecrust

Directions: Mix all the ingredients until smooth. Pour into piecrust and bake at 350 degrees for 45-60 minutes.

RASPBERRY CHOCOLATE CHEESECAKE: add ½ cup chopped frozen raspberries and chocolate chips (I usually use about ¼ cup) to cheesecake mixture before pouring into piecrust. Once cooled, drizzle melted chocolate on top.

JELLY SWIRL CHEESECAKE: once you pour the plain cheesecake mixture into your crust, but before you place it in the oven, swirl in a couple spoonfuls of your favorite jelly. Our favorites are cherry, raspberry, and strawberry.

CARAMEL CHOCOLATE CHIP PECAN TOPPING
- 1 cup pecans, chopped
- 3 TBSP butter, separated
- 3 TBSP sweetener

- 1/8 tsp vanilla extract
- 2 TBSP heavy cream
- ¼ tsp salt
- ½ cup chocolate chips

In a small saucepan melt 2 tbsp butter, sweetener, vanilla, and heavy cream. Let it bubble until golden brown (7 mins). Remove pan from heat and stir in the last tablespoon of butter. Mix in pecans. Pour pecan mixture over cooked cheesecake, press in chocolate chips. Chill in the fridge.

WORLD'S EASIEST COOKIES

Makes about 15 cookies.

Ingredients:
- 1 cup creamy peanut butter
- 1/2 cup powdered sweetener
- 1 egg

Directions: Combine all three ingredients into a bowl. Roll into balls, and then flatten with a fork. Bake for 10-13 minutes at 350 degrees. Store in an airtight container.

OATMEAL WITH VARIATIONS

Ingredients
- 1-2 cups old fashioned oats
- Almond or cashew milk

Directions: Place oats in a microwavable bowl, and add almond or cashew milk until oats are just barely covered—you don't want too much milk. Microwave for 1 ½ to 2 minutes.

BLUEBERRY MUFFIN: After removing oatmeal from the microwave, mix in vanilla Okios or Siggi's yogurt and 2-3 drops vanilla liquid stevia. Then sprinkle in a handful of blueberries, mix, and enjoy.

BANANA BREAD: After removing oatmeal from the microwave, mix in a banana-flavored Okios yogurt and some cinnamon. Cut up half a banana and mix it in. Enjoy your delicious breakfast!

Wilder Way Testimonials

What you're about to read are the true and unembellished testimonies from real women who have seen their health and their lives change by following my #WilderWay. These testimonies are why I do this! Thank you to each of these brave women for sharing their journey with us!

I've been on the #bgdir journey since January of 2016! I have to say it has been so life changing. I no longer stress about eating, and I never feel like I'm starving myself. I have the knowledge to take things one day and one meal at a time. No more anxiety about meal planning, I actually look forward to it. I have tried and have loved every Wilder Way recipe.

I can proudly say this is my happy life now. I am confident and proud to be me. I actually feel like a participant in life, and along the way I have had moments I never dreamed possible. I like being on an airplane now, and using the seat belt without an extender, and being able to put the table tray down. Score! I am not just watching as life passes by, I am trying new things and enjoying every minute. I have learned my body CAN move, and I thrive on the feeling of getting my sweat on. Jasinda and her passion and love for sharing this with us has changed my life. We are so lucky to be inspired by such an incredible woman. I am so proud to be a #wilderway gal for life. It is the best life! ~Donna K., Fabulous 40!

I would like to share a story with you. My husband, my two sisters, and I started this journey together. We love it, and it has been the best decision we have ever made. I share this program with people because it is a program that works.

I also would like to tell you about Heather; we talked online, and she wanted to know what I was doing for weight loss. That was in October, and now she is down 23 lbs and she will tell you it didn't feel like a diet. We message back and forth almost every day and have become friends. Really, I'm more like a mother to her. So if anyone is looking for a new way of life, this is the plan for you. Thanks again for all your information and for letting us bug you all the time! ~Carol K.

Reading Jasinda Wilder's books, following the plan, and doing the first 8-week Wilder Way Challenge in May of

2016 changed my life in ways I would never have imagined possible.

My first thoughts were "no sugar, no flour, no rice, and no potatoes? What is there left to eat? Okay…let's see if this is possible."

Over the next few weeks I learned so much about food, ingredients, and that there is a healthier and better option for all of your favourite meals! You don't miss out on anything! I learned to get my body moving outdoors! In public! In bright-coloured running sports gear! Joining a 5k!

OMG is this really me?

Yes, this is the new me! Self-confident! More energy! Healthier and happier!

And thanks to her mantras—slow and steady; listen to your body; give yourself grace; focus on the next meal; tomorrow is a new day—and the never-ending personal support through personal messages, live videos, and the FB group, nobody gets left behind! We lift each other up, stumble, and take detours sometimes, but we learn to get back on track, because we are worth it!

I could write on and on and never find the right words to do justice to the effects you as a person and your books have had on the lives of so many of us out there. You've invested so much time and energy and research, on top of being a mom of six and wife and author! You are like Ellen DeGeneres to me!!

Thank you so much Jasinda! And a big virtual hug from this German outpost #Wilderway girl! ~Monika S.

My cholesterol was high and I had just found out I was diabetic. I was in denial and ignoring the results. I went to an amusement park with my family and I couldn't fit on the rides. The look on my son's face was heartbreaking, and that was the push I needed to lose weight.

Your plan has been easy. I never knew that losing weight could be so easy! I used to drink at least 5 sodas a day. I gave them up within the first two weeks… even before I had to! I never thought I would be able to go a single day without soda, let alone 6 months. I went to the doctor and my cholesterol dropped 100 points and I am no longer diabetic. I lost 65 pounds in 6 months and I feel awesome! I can keep up with my kids and can't wait to go back to the amusement park and finally be able to ride the rides with my son! ~Lauren M., 32

April 2016: I remember it well because I knew something in my life had to change, but I didn't know how or where to start. Then I saw a FB post from Jasinda Wilder about a new book she had coming out about food and health. I had read a few of her fiction books, but didn't know much else about her. I was drawn to her for some reason, and I am so glad that I trusted my gut. In May 2016 I started on this new lifestyle journey and have never looked back.

To date I have lost and kept off 30 lbs! I know that might not seem like much, but it's gone and has been for almost 2 years. Thanks to that weight loss I have been off my blood pressure meds for over a year. I sleep well, my mind is clear and my doctor says I am getting healthier every day. My children are doing better in school than they ever have before and we are active instead of couch potatoes.

If you're looking for an easy and quick way to lose weight, this isn't the lifestyle for you, but if you're looking for a healthy and sustainable way to lose weight permanently, then come and join the #Wilderway. In addition to the book we have a *fabulous* FB group full of women and some men who are supportive, inspirational, and always there for you when you're ready to give up. Jasinda is also an AMAZING support and is always so encouraging, nonjudgmental, and she really does understand where you're at because she has been there too. I have had the pleasure of speaking with her a few times and each time she tells me she is proud of me. It brings tears to my eyes and makes me want to keep working harder. Through this journey Jasinda has taught me to love myself, and that it's okay to put myself first, which isn't easy for any mum out there to do. Thank you, Jasinda Wilder, for saving my family and me, and for getting us on the journey to being healthy and happy. ~Terra D.

My weight journey started in 2012. I was 152 lbs, and then my son Jacob passed away and I fell into a deep depression and gained almost 100 pounds. I was introduced to Jasinda's book in May of 2016 because I am a fan of her other books. I read it and immediately put into action the things she taught me. I also used the book as a guide in my home with my family and foster children.

Being a foster parent, we are challenged with many behaviors in children. I noticed right away that I was feeling better eating on the plan she created, and I started using it with the kids in my home as well. I noticed their behaviors changing, mental health improving, and the children were no longer as symptomatic of their diagnosed ailments and mental health. As behaviors changed, medications were lowered and, in some cases, discontinued with doctoral care. I am not a doctor, this is just my experience.

Myself, personally, I got my weight from 263 to 143 just following the plan and walking. I went from a size 26 jeans to a 12/14. I am not able to work out in the traditional manner due to a serious back injury that left me with 3 lbs of metal in my back that includes the hardware for a spinal cord stimulation unit. I am currently fused from my T11 to my S1 with screws and cages. So working out traditionally was not an option for me. But Jasinda's plan worked, and I noticed changes right away in the way I felt and the way that I started to look.

Fast forward to December 25th, 2017. My 18-year-old son Jarred passed away in a tragic accident and again I found myself in a depression and relying on the "meal train" from people to feed my family. I caught myself gaining back weight pretty quickly because I was eating what was brought to the house. It was easy, and I was just so thankful for everyone helping me with my huge family that I didn't even take into account what I was doing. We were just getting by, and I fell off the wagon. I am now sitting at 163 and am taking things a meal at a time and getting back where I was.

What I love about Jasinda's plan is that she doesn't advocate beating yourself up if you fall off the wagon. You simply get to the next meal and start over. There are many options for meals, snacks, fasting etc., so I was never hungry and I never felt like I was going without. My children now choose better options, and we notice right away that their behaviors change if they are given something that is against the plan. I could not have done it without her help and guidance. ~Angela D.

I have been overweight my whole life. I've tried dieting since I was a teenager (I'm 32 now) and could never stick to it. I would diet for a while and lose weight and then gain it all back plus some as soon as I started eating "normally." I lost around 30 lbs my senior year of high school and felt awesome. I kept the weight off during my first year of college and even lost a little more. I can't tell you the number of times I've heard how beautiful my hair is, but never how beautiful *I* was, because, of course, to most of the world, big women aren't beautiful. But eventually it was my turn and even though I was always the big friend, I was able to find love, and after being together for a few years we were blessed with a son.

Being happy and in love, I gained probably 60 lbs those

first few years. The pregnancy was rough because I was nauseated the whole time and threw up every meal I ate, so I only gained 18 lbs. In December of 2008, when I delivered my son via C-section, I weighed 299 lbs, my highest weight ever. It didn't bother me because I was riding a high of having my wonderful baby boy and being his mom. Eight weeks after I had my son, thanks to what I assume must be the effects of breastfeeding, I had my weight down to 266 lbs. I felt great and I was so happy.

During the first year of my son's life, I was so happy that I gained those 30 lbs back and I honestly don't know how much more. I refused to weigh myself, because I didn't want to know. I also didn't let people take pictures of anything but my face. I was ashamed of myself, but I didn't allow it to show. And I just kept eating. I was doing some exercising, but I was constantly eating.

Fast forward to 2016, March 2016 to be exact. My dad was diagnosed with end-stage renal disease and I wanted to be able to give him a kidney to help him live. I got the news from the doctor that I was probably the best candidate to do this, but I would have to lose weight before I could be considered for surgery. I was devastated but determined. The doctors said my dad could live on dialysis for 10-15 years, so I told myself that I would do this for him. I would lose weight so that I could keep my dad live. But, honestly, I was stuck in the same situation that I have always been in: needing to lose weight, and trying diets I couldn't stick to.

I was uninformed as far as proper nutrition went, and I

didn't understand my body at all. I had 2-3 headaches a week, at least one of them migraine strength. I stayed nauseated and threw up several times a week. I would overeat and it would be all the worst stuff. I was drinking 8-10 12oz cans of Pepsi or Mountain Dew a day. Yet I couldn't figure out why I stayed sick. I didn't realize I was literally killing myself.

Then one day I was on FB and saw a post from one of the authors I liked to read in the romance genre that was promoting a self-help type of book. As I looked into it, I could see she was changing things, and something just instantly clicked in me, and told me to order it. The book was called *You Can Do It*, by Jasinda Wilder. That was May of 2016. My weight at that time was 278 lbs, only down from before because I had married the love of my life in November 2015, so I had lost a little weight for the wedding. When I got Jasinda's book, I read it in one day.

My life changed instantly. I had talked two of my friends into ordering the book with me as a "let's do it together" support type of thing. So after they read it, very quickly I might add, one of the friends suggested we go the whole next day without soda. Remember, that was my drug of choice. I was an addict. I felt like I might die if I tried going without it, but I agreed. So I went the whole next day with no soda. That was a Wednesday. I felt so proud of myself that I could do it that I decided to see if I could go until Friday, and then Friday turned to the next day and the next, and now it's February 2018 and I've never looked back.

I know that isn't exactly the way the book lays out the

plan, but I had to read the book several more times to get a better grip on the actual concept of what Jasinda was talking about. So then I cut out all sugars and boy, did I see a difference in everything! By week eight, the headaches were few and far between, and my stomach issues were going so much better. My skin cleared up. As I was incorporating Jasinda's plan into my life, I realized that I had failed for so long because I honestly didn't know how to eat or exercise.

This book literally changed my whole way of living and it still inspires me and changes me every time I open it. I open it often because I'm always referring back as my body is changing, because my eating is changing too. Almost 2 years into this journey, I have lost 85 lbs and I don't know how many inches because I refused to take before pictures or measurements when I started because I honestly didn't think I could stick to this. I didn't want to be even more embarrassed when I quit again. I didn't have confidence in myself then.

I've lost weight, but I've also improved on so many other levels. I can physically do things I never could have before. My headaches are nonexistent. My stomach problems are gone. My skin looks better than it ever has. I've lost weight, but I've gained confidence and my health has improved. I did a 5K, and I didn't just walk it. I've never been more proud of myself, and when people ask how I did it I say two things: Prayer, and Jasinda's book. I still want to lose an additional 30 pounds, and I continue to strengthen and tone my body. I finally love my body and I'm working on taking care of it now. Finally! I hate that it took 31 years to do that. ~Shawna J.

"I will not quit!" I remember saying those words to myself when I made a promise to Jasinda Wilder when she literally saved my life.

I've come to realize it is truly not about the number on the scale, but about the way I feel both mentally and physically. The way my clothes fit, the things I do on a daily basis to challenge myself. It's my daily food choices and it's the feeling I get when I see myself in the mirror. Not only do I see a beautiful healthy glowing me, I now see a woman who has so much to be thankful for, and I've gained so much confidence as well. I'm finally taking control of my health; both my inner health and my outward appearance. Most of all, I got my life and health back. My mental clarity is so much better. I focus better. I feel stronger and I'm doing things I haven't done in over 30 years. This is one of the most amazing things I've ever been through in my life. Thank you Jasinda, from the bottom of my heart. ~Maria S.

In May of 2016, I weighed almost 250 lbs. I would get short of breath just walking out to get the mail. I was miserable in my own body. I read *You Can Do It* and started the program. Almost two years later, I'm down 100 lbs. I feel better than I ever have. The chronic pain I've dealt with for the last 20 years due to my excess weight is all but a memory. I never feel deprived. I'm active, and I'm finally living the life I never thought I would have. I honestly can't say thank you enough, or even begin to express how much I wish for everyone who is struggling, to go for it! You CAN Do It!! #WilderWayforLife ~Christina S.

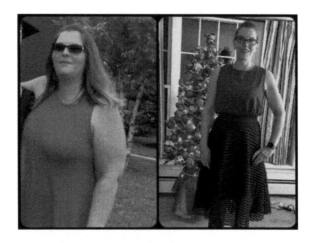

In May 2016 I read a Facebook post about a book Jasinda had coming out and a group that was going to do an eight-week challenge together. I was very overweight, in pain at all times, and had terrible insomnia. I was constantly exhausted, suffering terrible migraines, and had lost nearly half of my hair. I thought, "I have nothing to lose and I can do anything for eight weeks." I started the first day of the first challenge.

Over the course of nearly two years I have lost over eighty pounds and I've maintained that weight loss. I sleep like a baby and have more energy than I've ever had. I walk or hike an average of three to five miles a day, six to seven days a week. Between May 2015 and April 2016 I had fourteen migraines, but since starting the program I have an average of four per year! Sixty percent of my missing hair has grown back. I have much more confidence than I did before. Best of all, I am strong, I am healthy, and I am an active participant in my life. I am a work in progress. A huge thank you to Jasinda for giving me the tools to change my life. I will forever be grateful. ~Melissa R.

My journey began in 2015 when I discovered that I was hypothyroid and had Hashimoto's Thyroiditis. They also found out that I had thyroid cancer and I ended up having a total thyroidectomy. Over the course of five or six years, before these diagnoses, I gained about 70 lbs. I've been a lifetime member of Weight Watchers since 1984. Everything I did—eating "right" and exercising wasn't working for me.

In May of 2016, Jasinda Wilder published an amazing book, *You Can Do It*. Did I want to change my way of thinking about dieting and eating, and get healthier? How about the way I exercised? The answer was yes and I joined the first group after the beta testers.

I came to realize that my thyroid meds needed support. I began adding supplements and slowing removing sugar and white carbs from my diet. I was never a soda drinker and not much of a dessert eater, so the beginning process wasn't as hard for me, as it was for others. I began to notice that I was losing inches and my face was not as puffy. The numbers on the scale were moving slowing, but steadily, and I was down a size after a month. I'm a teacher of children between the ages of eighteen months and three years. One day, I wore a larger pair of shorts to school, without a belt. We were all surprised when one of my little girls pulled on my shorts and down they came! It became easier to breathe as the months passed. Also, my IBS is now in remission, I'm no longer prediabetic and my thyroid numbers are great. I'm down 45 pounds and four sizes. I've done a few 5K runs, and I continue to lift weights (and babies, lol). Friends, the love and support I've had from Jack and Jasinda Wilder, and the Wilder Way, has been priceless. ~Anne A.

FATS

nuts and nut butters
avocado
butter
cheese
cream
mayo
oils
whole eggs
full fat meats
chocolate
ice cream *
nut flour

*Bryers Carb Smart
and no sugar added coconut dream

Neutral Choices

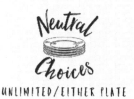

UNLIMITED/EITHER PLATE

spices
lemons & limes
berries
asparagus
broccoli
cabbage
cauliflower
celery
cucumber
egg plant
green beans
all greens
mushrooms
onions
peppers
sprouts
squash
tomatoes (salsa)
zucchini
Dreamfields pasta
Okios 000 yogurt
Low carb/Whole wheat
Mission wraps

CARBS/STARCHES

sprouted breads
sprouted cereal
blue corn chips
old fashioned oats
apples
apricots
bananas
grapes
kiwi
melon
oranges/tangerines
peaches
nectarines
pears
pineapple
plums
popcorn
quinoa
rice (brown, wild)
beans
hummus
lentils
carrots
corn
potatoes (sweet)
WASA crackers (4)

The three possible plates for your meal

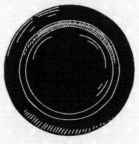

THE BLACK PLATE
Protein + Fat(s)

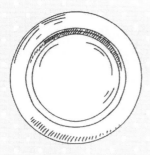

THE WHITE PLATE
Protein + Carbohydrates and starches

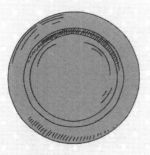

THE GRAY PLATE
Protein + Fat(s) + Carbohydrates/starches
(4-5 of these per week max)

To be informed of new releases, special offers, and other Jasinda news, sign up for Jasinda's email newsletter.

www.jasindawilder.com

www.biggirlsdoitrunning.com

My other health and wellness titles:

You Can Do It

You Can Do It Companion Journal

You Can Do It: Strength

RECIPE INDEX

Made in the USA
San Bernardino, CA
06 January 2019